All my longings lie
open before You,
O Lord; my sighing is
not hidden from You.
My heart pounds,
My strength fails me;
Even the light has
gone from my eyes.
~Psalm 38:9,10

Though You have
made me see troubles,
many and bitter, You
will restore my life again;
from the depths of the
earth You will
again bring me up.
~Psalm 71:20

Mosaic moments

Devotionals for the Chronically Ill

Lisa Copen & Friends

RMP

Rest Ministries Publishers
SAN DIEGO, CA

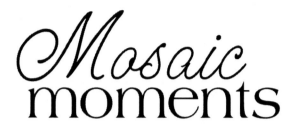

Mosaic Moments

ISBN: 0-9716600-3-4
Library of Congress Control Number: 2002096293

Request for information should be sent to:
Rest Ministries, Inc., a Christian organization
that serves people who live with chronic illness or pain.
P.O. Box 502928, San Diego, CA 92150
858-486-4685; Toll-free 888-751-REST (7378)
Web site: www.restministries.org
Email: rest@restministries.org
Please contact us for information on large-print editions.

Printed in the United States of America

"*Mosaic Moments* illustrates what people with hidden illnesses are becoming in the hands of God's workmanship. I must confess that their spiritual development, maturity, and insight are far ahead of mine." *Don Crooker, President of the Christian Council on Persons with Disabilities, International*

"There are times when chronic illness threatens to steal something new from every area of life. It is then that Rest Ministries has proven to be my lifeline, their daily devotionals I receive via e-mail providing manna for the moment. *Mosaic Moments* has stocked that manna in a single comforting compilation. A virtual cupboard brimming with heart-to-heart stories grounded in Biblical truth, it is written by real people in the trenches of chronic illness—people who deal with the very issues I face each day as I live with chronic pain caused by neurofibromatosis. I finished each serving not simply fulfilled, but encouraged to go on. *Mosaic Moments* is truly heaven's *Chicken Soup for the Chronically Ill Soul." Roberta Messner, Ph.D., R.N., author of numerous medical and inspirational articles on living with chronic pain; co-contributor to* Guideposts *and* Daily Guideposts

"In writing *The Art of Helping,* I realized that people are willing to rally around and provide support to their friends facing a short term crisis, but are much less willing to walk beside a friend facing a long-term long condition. As a part their support community, it is vital that we connect with and relate to our friends dealing with a chronic condition. *Mosaic Moments* provides such an opportunity. This beautiful devotional offers hope and reassurance that we are never alone. May we take these promises and apply them in our daily lives, not just as the one walking the path of chronic illness, but as their companion in the journey as well." Lauren Littauer Briggs, Author, *The Art of Helping — What to Say and Do When Someone is Hurting*

"Broken by the Potter, Lisa opens her heart and life to share with us what her loving Lord has taught her. *Mosaic Moments* is for anyone who has been broken and longs for a refreshing drink." *Lois A. Denier, Editor of* Jars of Clay

"These devotions are not empty morsels *promising* nutrition, but *real* meat from the Life Giver Himself for those so desperately needing spiritual sustenance. May God bless your work." *Darlene K. Hanson, Librarian for Polio Experience Network and a Horizon Hospice volunteer*

"I am so thankful to be able to offer *Mosaic Moments* as a resource to those who struggle with chronic pain and illness. Rarely are there words to convey my heartfelt concerns for suffering. With *Mosaic Moments* I am able to share a spiritual cup of cold water. It offers words of loving and caring I believe Jesus Himself would share." *Julie Russell, R.N., Parish Nurse, Stephen Minister*

"It's amazing! So many U-turns in this world involve the work of God's hand through illness, but it's often hard to see the end result when you are in pain. *Mosaic Moments* is a daily guidepost for those who are suffering, offering compassion, understanding, joy and even humor. Lisa and others become vulnerable to give a glimpse into their journey and what sustains them." *Allison Gappa Bottke,* author of *God Allows U-Turns series*

"The authors of *Mosaic Moments* prove that just because you have pain doesn't mean you have to be one. With joy flooding forth in concise bursts of truth and integrity, they write convincingly and hopefully. This book is written by those who know [pain] for those who know [pain]." *Phillip H. Barnhart, Doctor of Ministry, Founding Pastor and Pastor Emeritus of Chapel on the Hill, Lake Geneva, Wisconsin*

"I've always known that Rest Ministries is unique as it addresses the needs of those living with chronic pain and illness. *Mosaic Moments* is the best and most poignant resource I have read. It will fill a big need in the lives of those who live with pain and limitations every day of their lives. I will wholeheartedly recommend it to our readers." *Aubrey Beauchamp R.N., Editor of* A New Heart, *USA Hospital Christian Fellowship*

In Loving Memory
of my Grandmother
Austeen Griffin

She said, "I don't ask
God to heal me. I just
ask Him to let me walk
one more day. And
so far, He has."

Thank you for the legacy
that you left to me,
Grandma.

For Our Readers

"And the God of all grace, who called you to His eternal glory in Christ, after you have suffered a little while, will Himself restore you and make you strong, firm and steadfast," (1 Peter 5:10).

What you hold in your hand is nothing short of a miracle. Each devotional in this book is written by someone who lives with a chronic illness or with daily pain. They didn't live *through* it but rather they *are* living with it today. I typed the manuscript with six fingers because my right hand can barely bend. Many nights my hand cramped as I tried to hold the pen and edit. Other writers moved all over their homes, trying to find a comfortable seat in which to hear God's voice and let the words flow. Some wrote a paragraph over and over, frustrated that their cognitive abilities were not as quick as they were before illness. One man breathes with the help of a ventilator; the Holy Spirit overflows in His words.

We do not come to you with words of wisdom, as if we know all of the answers. Each day, we still endure doubts, insecurities, and questions about why God chose this particular path to use our abilities. Why, we ask, when we have a heart to serve, did He find it in His best interest to give us a set of limitations to overcome... or even work within? We may not have complete understanding, but we know who does: Jesus. Little by little, God is restoring us as He promises in 1 Peter 5:10.

So, with a heart to write, a calling to pick up the pen, and a prayer that God will somehow use our afflictions, we bring you this devotional book. We hope that you will be comforted in knowing that you are not alone. Maybe we can even shield you from experiencing a few of the lessons that we've had to learn the hard way. We pray that this book will bring you comfort during periods of despair, be a night-light of hope through sleepless nights, and that it will pull you through the nobody-understands-blues and the feelings of what-have-I-got-to-lose? Prepare to be restored!

Acknowledgements

Searching for Christian support since the onset of my illness in 1993, I began Rest Ministries in 1997. I scoured the Christian bookstores for a devotional book for people with illness, but I came up empty-handed. It was then that this book was born. In the meantime, Rest Ministries was growing quickly, and people were congregating at the Rest Ministries web site, becoming acquainted and encouraging one another to persevere and hold on to Christ.

One woman approached me and said, "We really need something positive each day, like a devotional."

"You are so right!" I told Kay DeCarlo. "I've been wanting to do this and have not had the time."

"Well, I'll do it. I'd be happy to," replied Kay.

That was years ago, and Kay, as our volunteer devotional coordinator, continues to send out devotionals each day to thousands of people. God has transformed the lives of many through our volunteers, all of whom have humbly stepped forward to assist with writing devotionals. Kay, I hope you know I never could have done this without you. You have administrative abilities that make me appear organized and you have a commitment that awes me. Most of all, you have a gift with words from the Holy Spirit and the ability to reach out to people right where they are hurting. Thank you will never be enough, but—thank you!

It's said, "God does not ask for our abilities, but our availability." Rest Ministries is blessed to have volunteers with both ability and availability, despite their own chronic conditions. Thank you for exposing your vulnerabilities to share how Christ fulfills you. You daily inspire me.

To list the people who have blessed my life through Rest Ministries would fill a book, but I hope you realize how deeply you are appreciated. Many volunteers have contributed countless hours—simply loving people who are hurting — that others have turned away. Anne, Jake, Patti,

Kat, Pamela, Trish, Ron, John, Cindy, Judy, LeeAnn, Rex, John, Shona, and many more—you are so precious in His sight. God knows how much you sacrifice to serve. Adriana Stavish, I could not have done this without you. Your editing skills, willingness to work around my crazy schedule, and your precious heart, made this book complete. Thank you.

To all who receive our daily devotionals online, your encouraging feedback keeps us going on days when we wonder if we can do life with illness a day longer. Without you, the chronic illness journey would be lonely and much cloudier. We may not want to vacation in Guam (see page 22), but with you along for the trip, it's been much more fun.

Thank you to two people I admire and whose books shaped my path on living with illness: Tim Hansel, author of *You Gotta Keep Dancin'*, the first book I was given on living with illness. Thanks, Tim, for saying, "Go for it." It made all the difference. To Joni Eareckson Tada, you didn't know me from anyone, and yet you made me feel like God had hand-chosen me for a ministry in which I felt most unequipped. Your encouragement was affirmation that God had a plan bigger than myself or my abilities. Your book, *When God Weeps,* put my beliefs into words so that I could share who God is with others who seek tangible answers upon which to cling.

To my spiritual mentor, Connie Kennemer: You make every woman who knows you feel like she is your best friend, but you are truly stuck with me. You have propelled me forward on this challenging, unpredictable path of ministry through the perfect combination of lattes and prayers. Your friendship has made ministry, writing, and even illness fun.

Loving thanks to my parents, Lloyd and Diane Safley, who always told me I could do anything and then raised me to believe it was true, so true that I ignorantly plowed ahead, thinking, "Of course I can write a book!" Special thanks to my sister, Michelle, to Mom, Ruth and Shayla for the giggles I will always treasure at Rest Ministries' exhibit escapades.

In loving memory of John Madrid, who would have looked at this book and said, "Wow. God is so awesome."

To my husband, Joel. . . none of this would exist without your unconditional support and daily encouragement. When I complain of pain, you never say, "Well, if you wouldn't sit at the computer so long. . . ." When dinner comes out of a box, you act just as enthused as when it's homemade. I always knew I loved you, but I never anticipated that loving you would be the thread that would connect so many of my dreams.

~*Lisa*

"But those who suffer, He
delivers in their suffering; He
speaks to them in their affliction."
Job 36:15

"For He has not despised or disdained
the suffering of the afflicted one; He has not
hidden His face from him, but has
listened to his cry for help."
Psalm 22:24

Introduction

I have recently taken up a long-anticipated hobby, mosaics. Mosaic is the art form of gluing tiles or pieces of broken dishes to anything one can imagine and then filling them with grout. The result is a beautiful piece of artwork, formed out of that which was originally meant for the trash.

Romans 9:21 says, "Does not the potter have the right to make out of the same lump of clay, some pottery for noble purposes and some for common use?" Our lives are so much like these common pots. God formed us from the beginning and has anticipated this lifetime that we would spend on earth. He knew in advance that you would be sitting right where you are today, reading this very book. Before our illness, like a commonly used platter, we all served. Some of us served the Lord, while others of us served the world. Either way, one day we all felt a "smash!"

Our illness splintered our lives into many pieces. A few of the fragments—perhaps spouses, children, jobs, independence, and self-confidence were lost in the process. Looking around at the pieces of broken pottery, it seemed that our usefulness was gone; it disintegrated in front of our very eyes. We believed we would never be able to serve anyone or any purpose again. Some of us are experiencing this feeling right now. *What can God do with this broken body? What is His purpose for my life now? I could serve Him so much better without this distraction of pain!* Even those of us who are past this grief stage still find ourselves edging up to these thoughts, wondering and waiting. *When will God show me my new purpose? Why is His timing always so much longer than my own? I want to serve God, but how can I when I feel so poorly?*

Despite the lack of evidence that we may have that God is actively involved in our lives, right at this moment, He is; He is sorting through the fragments, the pieces of your common pot, and He is creating a magnificent piece of art. In the book of Job, we find Job attacked over and over with trauma and loss. He withstands it all, looking towards God, with faith that He will restore him and his life for His glory. Then Satan takes action that, in Job's viewpoint, is the final straw. Satan afflicts Job "with painful sores from the soles of his feet to the top of his head," (Job 2:7). How does Job react? Does he get mad? Cry? No. "Then Job took a piece of broken pottery and scraped himself with it as he sat among the ashes," (Job 2:8). Physically weak from disease and the emotional suffering, Job probably collapsed. Sitting in the ashes, he looked over at a piece of broken pottery, probably one of the few remainders and reminders of all he had owned days earlier. He picked it up, looked at the dirt on it, and then started to pick at his sores, using it as a tool.

There are theories about Job's actions. Surely, he realized he would likely cause infection; perhaps he just wanted to end his life, wondering if life was worth fighting for if God wasn't going to intervene when he needed Him the most. Maybe he was numb, sitting on the ground, trying to remember how he had gotten into this messy situation. Perhaps, he was angry with God and trying to hold his emotions back before he exploded. Whatever the reason, we can assume that Job was downtrodden and felt he may as well sit in the ashes, as his body was likely returning to them soon.

How often we feel broken, like David, the author of the Psalms. "I am forgotten by them as though I were dead; I have become like broken pottery," (Psalm 31:12). Though we do not know God's purpose, we can find peace in knowing He has one and that He always remains in control. God predicted that, in this world that contains sin, we would become broken souls without Him. "It will break in pieces like pottery, shattered so mercilessly that among its pieces not a fragment will be found for taking coals from a hearth or scooping water out of a cistern," (Isaiah 30:14).

Do you feel that your life has been smashed to pieces for no apparent reason? I think all of us who live with any kind of physical ailment have felt abandoned at one time or another

—sometimes for years! You are not alone in your wonders and worries. Even those who have known the Lord for many years, question God's motives in "destroying" their lives through illness. During Biblical times, Job asked, "Why have You made me Your target? Have I become a burden to You?" (Job. 7:20b). David pleas, "O Lord, do not rebuke me in Your anger or discipline me in Your wrath. For Your arrows have pierced me, and Your hand has come down upon me. Because of Your wrath there is no health in my body," (Psalm 38:1-3a). In reading your Bible you will find that many people questioned God about His reasons for their sufferings. Little has changed through the centuries. We still want to know why.

What you will find in this book is a group of people who live with various forms of chronic illness, facing affliction and pain every day of their lives. Although we still have the ailments, we also have the answer: the Lord Jesus Christ. None of us can comprehend facing each morning without the assurance that the Lord knows what He is doing. We each believe that, despite the quietness of God at times, He is active in our lives and that we have no reason to doubt His everlasting love. In Isaiah 29:16, the Lord says, "You turn things upside down, as if the potter were thought to be like the clay! Shall what is formed, say to Him, who formed it, 'He did not make me?' Can the pot say of the potter, 'He knows nothing'"? Truly, we are reminded daily, we know nothing. All that we once put our faith in, such as our health or careers, was taken away in an instant when our bodies rebelled. When illness crashes into your life, there is nowhere left to put your faith but in the Lord.

Ken Hutcherson, a professional football player turned pastor, says, "I've always admired 'tea kettle' Christians. They can be up to their necks in hot water and still sing! The world wants to know how this God you talk about makes a difference in your life when you're sitting on the burner. They want to see the reality of a life within you beyond anything they've ever experienced."[1] Well, friends, we're on the burner, the heat is on, and it is time for us to decide what tune we're going to sing. The only reason we can do this, with faith that God's purpose will prevail, is because He promises us. "Like clay in the hand of the potter, so are you in my hand," (Jeremiah 18:6).

God has the grout ready. We are in His hands. He wants to pattern your broken pottery pieces into a mosaic that will glorify Him. No plain old terra-cotta plant holder for your life! You're going to be something special, something that adorns Him. He is making something *noble.*

It is easy to believe that God was holding us in His hands, tripped, and hollered, "Oops!" as our life flew from His grasp, out of His control. How can this life we lead be His true intention when we feel like we've been dropped? Because God doesn't do things logically. Those who give everything away are the wealthiest; those that give away their lives are eternally saved, (see Matthew 19:30). Those that allow themselves to be cracked pots will be God's masterpieces. Regardless of what your circumstances are right now, I can say with conviction: God is not fumbling around in heaven, trying to make something miraculous out of His mess; He's not trying to design something opulent out of His "oops."

Job suffered great loss and immense sorrow, but not a moment of it was the result of God's lack of control. Remember this: God is *always* in control. Perhaps, with tears in His eyes, He held the hammer that broke your world apart—knowing that in the end, He would piece it back together. For Job, "The Lord blessed the latter part of Job's life more than the first," (Job 42:12). God wants to make you Christ-like; He is making you noble. He is moving you off that discount-shelf kind of life that you were living and preparing you for something grander. He will bless the latter part of your life and restore the years that you have lost. "I will repay you for the years the locusts have eaten," says the Lord, (Job 2:25). Anticipate it. Put your joy in it. Have faith.

It's hard to comprehend, but through the loss of your health, you will someday look back and see that you were blessed more after the loss than before the loss. Ephesians 3:20 says, "Now to Him who is able to do immeasurably more than all we ask or imagine, according to His power that is at work within us. . . ." How can God bless us in this mess? Because He gives more than we can possibly ask or imagine—sometimes more pain, *always* more joy. We will come to realize that it is not a peace or joy that we could have designed, because logically it's impossible to be happy within the circumstances in which we live. It seems a bit odd. It's not the way we expected to find God's blessings.

"I will give you the treasures of darkness, riches stored in secret places, so that you may know that I am the Lord," (Isaiah 45:3). When you know the Savior, somehow, it all makes sense.

I Miss It!

"I tell you the truth, you will weep and mourn while the world rejoices. You will grieve, but your grief will turn to joy," (John 16:20).

I stood at church in deep pain during worship; finally, I self-consciously sat down when standing became unbearable. The next chorus lyrics began, ". . .with God. . . I can stand in spite of pain." *Lo – o – rd!* I whispered up. *Come on! I feel weird enough sitting. Can I have a break?* I whispered to my husband about the irony of the lyrics. "It's symbolism," he said with a smile. I knew that, but the timing of the song was ironic.

I miss standing for worship. I miss being able to clap. My wrists don't turn; my hands don't move normally. I miss the power in my lungs that can lift a strong voice to the Lord. Life has brought the need to compromise and improvise, but there are still things I miss. I miss weird things, like sitting on the floor, knocking on a door, or carrying something with confidence that it won't drop. I miss long journeys in the car and going on rides at the fair. I miss spontaneity. I miss the absence of pain, the silent and unconscious void of hurting.

The Apostle John knew we would experience this. He knew in advance that believers would weep and mourn while the world rejoiced. God always knew that, while nineteen-year-old girls screamed over boy bands, my soul would weep to simply be able to stand and praise my God. While thirty-something women would rarely see their children because they chose careers, my soul would weep over waiting for the blessing of a child. Life isn't fair, but it will turn… to joy! "I am greatly encouraged; in all our troubles my joy knows no bounds," (2 Corinthians 7:4).

God, I have hope and confidence because You promise joy—not just "better days" or tastes of happiness, but pure and simple joy. I trust You will deliver because You never fail. I am weak, but You are strong. Yes, Jesus loves me! ~*Lisa Copen*

I Will Have What She's Having

"Now I rejoice in what was suffered for you, and I fill up in my flesh what is still lacking in regard to Christ's afflictions, for the sake of His body, which is the church," (Colossians 1:24).

After months of pain, I decided to try acupuncture. After the needles were inserted, the acupuncturist left me lying uncomfortably on a hard surface, and I heard him enter the room next door to begin the assessment of a new patient. "I'm here to increase my metabolism," she explained, and he told her what he could offer for her quest to lose weight. I couldn't move, or I would have jumped up and hollered, "I'll have what she's having!" A few more needles couldn't hurt!

Despite the fact that we live in constant pain, each day in which we glorify God, within our circumstances, we are a *more* effective witness for Christ than if we had been healed. That can be a painful thing to hear. Joni Eareckson Tada, Christian author and quadriplegic, shares that, when she gets into an elevator with strangers and they are held captive, she sings *Amazing Grace* until she reaches her floor. She wants to leave people wondering, "What is it that makes that woman in a wheelchair sing *Amazing Grace?"*[2] Would they be so intrigued if she walked?

Do people look at you and say, "I'll have what she's having! I want what he has"? Even as I wanted to shout this out to the acupuncturist, I knew it would cause more pain; yet I saw the end result as worthwhile. Through our illness, God can make us a living example of what He offers to those who hurt. Through Him, all the good things of life are still possible—joy, not just happiness; fellowship, not just friends. God knows how to explicitly weave together the infirmities that we experience; He turns the sins of the world into His recruiting crusades for the souls of those around us.

It's not easy, Lord. Help me to make the choice each morning to let the day be a sacrifice of praise; I trust it's worth it! *~Lisa Copen*

Are They Right About My Faith?

"All my friends are waiting for me to slip," (Jeremiah 20:10). "You have taken my companions and loved ones from me; the darkness is my closest friend," (Psalm 88:18).

"If you only had faith, then you would be well. Don't you believe in the power of prayer and that God does not want you to be sick?" Do these words sound familiar? Well-intentioned friends, family, or people at church offer their opinions. "You are sick because deep inside, you don't completely trust God to heal you!" This just isn't true. There are three types of healing: physical, emotional, and spiritual healing. God may choose to instantaneously heal us physically; however, He does not always work in the fast-paced ways that we desire. Sometimes, when it feels like we are flailing, we are in the center of God's will. Being obedient to Him is never an easy path to take, but it is so rewarding.

Have you noticed the different answers He provides to prayer requests? Sometimes the answer is, "Yes" or "Wait." Occasionally, God just says, "No." We'll always find people who feel that we don't have the faith to completely trust God. Jesus said, "If you have the faith the size of a mustard seed, nothing [will] be impossible for you," (Matthew 17:20).

When you are subjected to opinions, look toward Jesus. He was in constant prayer with His Father God, yet He suffered the rejection of men who didn't believe He was the Son of God; they nailed Him to a cross. "Peace I leave with you; my peace I give you. I do not give to you as the world gives. Do not let your hearts be troubled, and do not be afraid," (John 14:27). His answers won't always seem logical to those around us. God has a purpose for your suffering.

Lord, I have faith that You will answer my prayers one day at a time. Even when others doubt my faith, You know my heart. You know the size of the mustard seed. I believe I do have enough faith.

~Kay DeCarlo

I Feel Deported

"How can we sing the songs of the Lord while in a foreign land?" (Psalm 137:4).

There is a simple story that some use to explain what it feels like to be diagnosed with a chronic illness. Imagine for a moment that you have spent your entire life planning the perfect vacation to Paris. You have spent years learning to speak fluent French. You have acquired a taste for the exquisite food. You have studied the culture, the history, and have made specific plans of what you will do and see once you arrive. You have purchased new luggage and packed your bags for the appropriate weather. At last the day comes when your dreams will become reality. When the plane lands, however, the captain says, "Welcome to Guam. Please enjoy your stay, as there are no returning flights."

"What?" you scream! "This can't be! I'm supposed to be going to Paris. I prepared to visit France for years. I don't know anything about Guam! I refuse to get off this plane." "Sorry," says the captain. "This is your new home. You'll get used to it in time. You'll forget about Paris, France."

This is how it feels to be diagnosed with a chronic illness. You have spent your entire life assuming that you would be healthy or that any health problems that would occur would be curable. Then one day you realize you are in a different world. You must learn the language, the culture, everything, because there is no way to return to being the exact person you were before the illness.

I wonder if this is how David felt when he wrote, "How can we sing the songs of the Lord while in a foreign land?" (Psalm 137:4). Remember, however, "The Lord appeared to me in a faraway place…" (Jeremiah 31:3).

God, You never leave us. You're even more visible in the valleys than on the vacations if I search You out. ~*Lisa Copen*

The Compassion Factor

"Praise be to the God and Father of our Lord Jesus Christ, the Father of compassion and the God of all comfort, who comforts us in all our troubles, so that we can comfort those in any trouble with the comfort we ourselves have received from God," (2 Corinthians 1:3-4).

Before I started suffering with chronic nerve disease, I seldom had an ache. I taught elementary school for years without missing a day of work. When I retired, I had over a year of sick leave, and I could easily jog eight miles a day.

I will admit that I didn't have much compassion for the chronically ill. If someone had the flu or had been in an accident, I might understand for someone to complain a bit, but for one to complain for months of pain was difficult for me to understand. I would think, "It's mostly in her head" or, "If he would just get involved in something and get his mind off of himself, he would be just fine."

After coping with chronic pain for six years, my compassion for those dealing with pain and illness has greatly increased. As I have turned to God for comfort, I have also learned how to comfort others who are suffering. None of us would choose pain and illness, but perhaps it is a blessing in disguise.

Psalm 147:3 says, "He heals the brokenhearted and binds up their wounds." As we cope with pain, one of our greatest blessings will be our ability to reach out to others who are hurting, offering understanding comfort. In doing so, we can find purpose in our pain.

Lord, remind me to reach out to others, even in little ways. A kind word, a telephone call, a card, or a prayer are small gestures that make a big difference in the life of one who is suffering and discouraged.

~Patricia Armstrong

Sometimes I Don't Want to Pray

"The Lord is close to the brokenhearted and saves those who are crushed in spirit," (Psalm 34:18).

There are days when the heaviness of heart just won't go away. Often I am blessed with comfort from God, but occasionally I just don't feel like praying. I don't feel like praising God. I just want to be alone and curl inward. Depression can make one feel trapped in a pit of emotions that trigger insecurities, fear, and sadness. Alone, it can be devastating, but when one's body is unable to function effectively, it adds to the weight of our mental state. Even one of history's greatest preachers, Charles Spurgeon, said, "I am the subject of depression of spirit so fearful that I hope none of you ever get to such extremes of wretchedness as I go to."[3]

Psalm 34:18 promises that, "The Lord is close to the brokenhearted and saves those who are crushed in spirit." Chronic illness has a way of breaking one's heart and crushing one's spirit. There is so much loss associated with illness: loss of abilities, loss of friends, loss of dreams. It is hard for one's spirit *not* to become crushed over time. God promises, however, that this is one of those times that He will wrap His arms around us and make it all better. He doesn't offer a bandage, filled with only temporary relief, but rather a healing salve that will slowly mend our spirit and renew it.

Because of Jesus' sacrifice, no matter how hard I push God away, He will always remain nearby, just waiting for me to reach out to Him again. Many people believe that Christians shouldn't become depressed. They believe that depression is a sign that we lack faith; if we would open our Bible, we would feel better. Christians do get depressed, but the difference is that we can find hope outside of ourselves.

God, You understand that the world can have a way of crushing my spirit, and You promise, especially in these moments, to continue to be beside me and see me through the dark valley. *~Lisa Copen*

Living As A Broken Vessel

"Then Ananias went to the house and entered it. Placing his hands on Saul, he said, 'Brother Saul, the Lord, Jesus, who appeared to you on the road as you were coming here, has sent me so that you may see again and be filled with the Holy Spirit,'" (Acts 9:17).

I am convinced that many people are unable to truly find God until they are broken. As grueling as it is for us to hear, God breaks us, then remakes us as vessels that are fit for His purposes. Even Exodus 4:11 says, "The Lord said to him, 'Who gave man his mouth? Who makes him deaf or mute? Who gives him sight or makes him blind? Is it not I, the Lord?'" The Apostle Paul did not recognize who the Lord Jesus was until he was struck blind. Throughout the Bible, we see that it often takes a crisis before people will call on the Lord God for help. What about those of us, however, who already knew the Lord, are following Him, and yet we are still stricken with an affliction? We must realize that hardship comes to Christians not to make us believe in a God we already trust, but to make us more like the God that we trust.

Tim Hansel, author of *You Gotta Keep Dancin'*, says, "I finally came to the realization that if the Lord could use this body better the way it is, then that's the way it should be."[4] When the world would understand us if we cursed our circumstances and yet we offer blessings; when we should complain but we praise—these are the times we demonstrate who we are and the characteristics of God's love.

We aren't facing lions in Rome. We are His vessels. We are living in affliction and praising God in spite of it. God loves people; He adores us. He is patient, generous, and merciful. He treats people with loving kindness, even those that treat Him poorly. He is perfect, but we are not; we only become more like Him and prove who we are by the way we act.

Lord, help me remember nothing reflects You in my life better than my hopefulness in difficult circumstances. *~Karlton Douglas*

Learning To Rest

"By the seventh day God had finished the work He had been doing; so on the seventh day He rested from all His work," (Genesis 2:2).

I am attempting to learn how to rest. It may sound odd for a chronically ill person to have this as a personal goal, but last month I was convicted that I was stressing out too much about what needed to be accomplished. We each cope with illness in the best way we know how. For me, that involves keeping myself busy to distract myself from the pain. But the extreme busyness can cause more pain, and I end up going in circles. I pay a price and become frustrated with my continual mishaps of learning my limitations.

I don't allow myself to get depressed—a good thing, some may say, but not necessarily. When we are at our darkest moments, we reach out for God, ask for His strength, and say, "I can't do this without You, Lord!" When we rely solely on ourselves and refuse to have those dark moments, we miss out on what truly surrendering our hearts to God is all about.

When people tell me, "Go take a nap," I laugh and respond, "I'll take a nap when I fall over." But as I try to learn how to rest, both mentally and physically, I have taken a second look at rest. Even God rested. God didn't *need* to rest. He's God! He could have created the heavens and the earth and never taken a fifteen-minute break. But He *chose* to rest. He knew that resting was a priority for our lives and that He needed to set an example for us to follow.

Some friends believe that those of us with illness sit around lazily. They taunt us with how lucky we are to sleep in and not work. But rest is not a luxury. Rest isn't even a priority. It is a commandment. "Observe my Sabbaths and have reverence for my sanctuary. I am the Lord," (Leviticus 19:30).

Lord, help me honor this commandment and not think of it as a suggestion, but rather to make it a priority. *~Lisa Copen*

Seeking God's Face

"God is the strength of my heart and my portion forever," (Psalm 73:26).

I could almost see the face of God on that day. It was a day I sensed evil coming against me. When we battle daily with pain or illness, we sometimes feel like the evil one is coming against us, discouraging and depressing our soul.

I was having a physically painful day, and then I discovered that someone in my town was slandering me. As I sat weeping, God spoke to me. "See that you do not look down on one of these little ones. For I tell you that their angels in heaven always see the face of my Father in heaven," (Matthew 18:10).

Suddenly, I envisioned my Heavenly Father's face. What I saw was the utmost of Holy love, tenderness, gentleness, and softness as He looked at me. All of a sudden, all was well, and I did not sense evil coming against me any longer. I knew that ultimately nothing could harm me when that face belongs to my Heavenly Father.

Someday, all will be well with us. Soon, we will be gazing at His face, and we will have perfect health, peace, and joy, with no evil coming against us. We will never have another painful or weary day. Let us begin gazing on that face today; let Him speak His words of encouragement and love to us. "Other men see only a hopeless end, but the Christian rejoices in an endless hope," (Gilbert M. Beeken).[5] He has a purpose and a plan for our lives—just as they are. The next time someone speaks ill of us, let us remember our Father's beautiful face gazing upon us in holy love.

"Whom have I in heaven but You? And earth has nothing I desire besides You. My flesh and my heart may fail, but God is the strength of my heart and my portion forever," (Psalm 73:25-26).

~Virginia Ganskie

Create A Party In Your Pocket

"Has anyone planted a vineyard and not begun to enjoy it? Let him go home, or he may die in battle and someone else enjoy it," (Deuteronomy 20:6).

Friends think I am starting to get a bit silly. Our world is full of war and uncertainty, leaving many feeling weary and heavily burdened with concern and fear. Even the television refuses to allow us to escape, as dramas of crimes and gore are written for "our viewing pleasure."

In rebellion against this evil, I've decided to start seeing things through the eyes of a child. I've put aside my conservative, rational, boring self and am focusing on creating my own moments of joy, regardless of how silly they seem. I decorate with red pillows year-round (to the horror of one shopper, who said red was for Christmas!) I bought a faux-fur-covered notepad for my purse and found a pen that looks like a miniature doll fixed on an ink cartridge. I want more moments of instantaneous laughter in my life and more reasons to smile. I want "pockets of parties" to surround me to keep me focused on the joy that God provides, no matter how small. I need a bit of silliness to stay sane.

There will be moments of hurt and confusion; we may doubt that we will ever experience joy again. But during these moments, we may still numbly plant our vineyards— and then never enjoy them! Illness isn't fun. Unless we seek to create pockets of parties, there won't be laughs during the longings or pleasures while getting through the pain.

So the next time you smile at something and think, "No, that's way too silly. . ." say yes! Play with your kid's putty in the waiting room. Get crayons. Buy a fun hat. Wear the hot-pink scarf that someone gave you as a gag gift. Live a little.

Teach me how to enjoy the vineyard, God, that You have blessed me with this season.
~Lisa Copen

Woe To Me!

"Woe to me because of my injury! My wound is incurable! Yet I said to myself, 'This is my sickness, and I must endure it,'" (Jeremiah 10:1).

Two years ago, as my husband celebrated a birthday, he realized he was quickly beginning to approach the age of forty. "I need to do something to get in shape," he said.

"Try bicycling," I suggested. Within a week, he had bought a used bicycle, and, influenced from a stack of bicycling magazines, he quickly lost his reluctance to wear the bright apparel. Along with his new boost of health, equipment, and clothing, however, came overuse injuries.

I am quick to empathize with others who suffer with chronic illness. Fatigue, pain, side-effects of medication, and new disabilities are easy for me to relate with, and I give full compassion. When my healthy husband, however, rides his bike down the hill at forty miles an hour and then complains about the pain in his knees, my empathy wanes. An embarrassing sense of amusement crosses my emotions. As he complains about the clicking in his knee, I smile and utter, "Yep, I understand. I know just what you're talking about."

He went to physical therapy. He did his exercises. His pain is going away. Regardless of what I do to try to stop the degeneration in my joints from rheumatoid arthritis, it will only become worse. I'm envious. Each heart has its own hurt. Whatever affects one's life the most is deemed most important to that person. One will always see his pain as worse than mine because it's *his* own pain; my pain will always feel worse than others because it's *my* pain. It is times like this that I must lift up my jealousy to the Lord and quit comparing notes on who hurts worse.

Lord, help me be kind, gentle, and understanding. I don't want to think only of myself. Teach me compassion and empathy for all because, to You, everyone's hurts count equally. ~*Lisa Copen*

Trying Friends Can Try Our Emotions

"Have I ever said, 'Give something on my behalf, pay a ransom for me from your wealth?'" (Job 6:22).

Have you ever had a friend who desperately wanted to encourage you but who went about it all wrong? Good intentions may have been at the heart of the effort, but perhaps the words broke your heart rather than mended it. Many of us have heard, "If you aren't going to take my advice, you can't be that sick!"

Abraham Lincoln said, "When I am getting ready to reason with a man, I spend one-third of my time thinking about myself and what I am going to say and two-thirds about him and what he is going to say." Job's friends came with intentions of encouraging, yet they gave advice based on *their* understanding of the circumstances, not God's. In chapter six, Job reacts. "Hey! If you came to encourage me, then do it, but I don't need a lecture. I haven't asked you to fix anything, for a loan to rebuild, or for a piglet. I haven't asked you to go to the home improvement store, to borrow your maid, or even to bring me lunch. All I need is someone to listen." (My paraphrasing, obviously.)

Friends' advice can trouble us. I've wanted to say, "Look! Have I asked you to bring me dinner? Shared the burden of my finances? Have I endlessly complained about the pain? No. So just let me cry for a bit without offering any advice." Proverbs 15:1 says, "A gentle answer turns away wrath, but a harsh word stirs up anger." When we're tempted to make a list of the things our friends are doing wrong, we must remember this: They are doing the best they can within the boundaries of their experiences. They have human understanding, not the wisdom of our Father.

Lord, help me to be gentle with friends that don't fully "get it." You get it, God. Let me rely on You fully and be nice to my friends so I can show them You, Lord. *~Lisa Copen*

The Benefits Of Loss

"Whatever was to my profit I now consider loss for the sake of Christ. What is more, I consider everything a loss compared to the surpassing greatness of knowing Christ Jesus my Lord, for whose sake I have lost all things," (Philippians 3:7-8a).

What a shock when I suddenly became ill and found my life changing. First, and most importantly, I lost my independence. Soon, my husband left our marriage. I lost my ability to earn even a small income to augment my welfare benefit. Since I could no longer drive, I sold my car. Confined to home, I lost the fellowship of being part of my church and the ability to worship with others, even the pleasure of doing my own shopping. I can't travel, escape to the beach, or take a walk, and there's more.... Oh, I've lost so much that others take for granted! Perhaps you have lost even more than me.

Nevertheless, none of these things matter as long as I don't lose my relationship with Jesus Christ, for He is my reason for life itself. I struggled when my husband left, thinking I'd never cope on my own. One day, however, the Lord showed me that, although I could live without my husband, I could never live without Him. God promised He'd never leave me, and He has proved Himself faithful regardless of what I'm going through. Tim Hansel writes in *You Gotta Keep Dancin'*, "What a test adversity is. It can either destroy or build up, depending on our chosen response. Pain can either make us better or bitter."[6]

Each time I've lost another ability, I've grieved for it, but I have always been strengthened and comforted by Jesus, who understands everything I feel and experience. I've lost plenty, but I have gained much more by knowing my Lord in a deeper way. As Paul says, nothing surpasses the greatness of knowing Him.

As I lose my independence, Lord, and must depend more closely on You, help me find the hidden blessings. *~Janice McLaren*

Thankful For The Blooms

"Thanks be to God for His indescribable gift!" (2 Corinthians 9:15).

"You have jade plants!" my mom exclaimed. My husband and I had just moved into our home, and my parents came to assist. Mom was quickly investigating the yard. "They are huge! There is one out in the backyard and three in large containers that we can move onto the patio."

"What's a jade plant?" I said, showing my horticultural ignorance as a previous apartment-renter.

"They are beautiful plants, and Mrs. Ray used to love them. They're worth a lot too!"

Well! They were of value, but they were also sentimentally significant. Mrs. Ray was a neighbor we lived near during my childhood, who was like a grandmother to me. I had a connection with something she loved. It made them special. In December, small buds began to appear, and soon, the jade plants were covered with white flowers. I called my mom. "They're blooming," I said. "I didn't know they bloomed."

"Really? Oh, do you know how rare that is? Mrs. Ray used to be so excited when they would bloom. It takes years before they bloom." Had I not known this, I would not have appreciated the blooms. My jade plants, viewed from my office and kitchen windows, bring me great joy. The December blooms are heaven-sent, a small gift. It is one small indescribable gift for today.

Anne Frank once wrote, "I don't think of all the misery, but the beauty that still remains."[7] God asks us to "Give thanks to [Him], for He is good; His love endures forever," (Psalm 107:1). We must choose our joys one moment at a time.

Lord, You've surrounded me with indescribable gifts, but sometimes I must have someone point them out to me or search for them myself, as I don't realize the blooms are rare or something to be treasured. The less I understand life, the more I should seek to enjoy it.

~Lisa Copen

Learning How To Fish

"'I'm going out to fish,' Simon Peter told them, and they said, 'We'll go with you.' So they went out and got into the boat, but that night they caught nothing," (John 21:3).

A patient father, with enthusiasm for my sister and I to have the thrill of catching a fish, Dad would put the worm on the hook and hand us our poles. We would immediately place the pole into the pole holder and grab a magazine or a snack. Soon the lines would become tangled. We'd holler, "Dad! We need help!" Dad rarely had time to get his own line into the water and have that relaxing moment of just waiting for the fish. So often, we caught nothing.

Years later, my college roommate and I would grab her poles and waders and go to the river to flyfish. The men watched us blondes with curious skepticism as we got out the tackle box. "What are they biting?" Shari would ask, and they'd laugh until she started reeling in fish. I didn't catch many fish then either, but I did cast my line, and I got a nice tan.

Many times in our lives, we will cast our lines and wait. The patience required to see if God is going to heal us, provide financially, or give us the desires of our heart can seem unbearable and discouraging. Regardless of how skilled we are as fishermen, we may not catch any of the "answers" that we seek, but we still must learn how to enjoy the practice of fishing. What kind of fishing do you prefer?

Rest Ministries is an example of how I like to constantly "cast a line" and reel it in to see what is on the end. Then I cast again. Perhaps you are a fisherman who prefers to troll, praying and waiting patiently for God's response.

Father, life is full of opportunities for contentment, whether I am waiting or casting. Help me learn to enjoy the practice of fishing. Don't allow me to "read the magazines" and let You do all of the work. *~Lisa Copen*

Strengthened For The Battle

"Elijah came to a broom tree, sat down under it and prayed that he might die. 'I have had enough, Lord' he said. 'Take my life,'" (1 Kings 19:4).

Elijah was worn out. He had served God for many years in the face of great hardship. Now the wicked Queen Jezebel had ordered him killed. Exhausted, the prophet wanted God to remove him from the struggle. God didn't. Instead, He strengthened Elijah and sent him out to continue the battle.

Those of us who suffer with debilitating chronic illnesses can understand how Elijah felt. I, too, have asked God to take me home to Him when I have felt too weary to continue. One night I had a dream that encouraged me greatly. In it, I was standing on the bank of a wide, tempestuous river. I wanted to reach my parents' home on the opposite side, but the water was flowing quickly, and I am not a strong swimmer.

In my dream, I decided that I would simply walk across the water as Jesus had done. I stepped out. I sank like a stone. The water was over my head, and I couldn't breathe. I was drowning. Terrified, I shoved one hand up out of the water and gasped, "Jesus!" Suddenly, I felt a strong hand grasp mine. I knew that it was Jesus. I expected Him to lift me out of the water and set me safely on the far shore. But to my surprise, He stepped down into the water beside me, and together, Jesus and I walked along the riverbed. We were completely submerged, but I was able to breathe as if on dry land. When we reached the other side, I stepped safely on to the shore. This dream made me realize that Jesus might not always lift me out of my problems, but He will always walk through them with me.

Lord, like Elijah, I may ask You to end my struggles, and You may refuse. But, like Elijah, I can count on You to give me the strength to carry on. *~Mary Lou Cornish*

God Knows Tired

"Jesus was tired from His journey and sat down by the well," (John 4:6).

One of the most often-told Bible stories is of Jesus talking with the Samaritan woman at the well. She became a believer and left her hometown to follow Jesus. Her shared testimony brought many people to God. How did Jesus meet this woman? "Jesus was tired from His journey and sat down by the well," (John 4:6).

It is a comfort to me that even Jesus, Lord of all Lords, became tired. He simply wanted to sit down and rest for a moment. He wanted to have a drink of water so that He could feel refreshed and continue on His journey. God had other plans. God knew that, although Jesus was fatigued, in the next few minutes Jesus would meet a young woman; she would follow Jesus, become a disciple, and her testimony would transform many lives for years to come, bringing people to know God's salvation.

When we grow tired and wonder how God can possibly use our bodies, remember how God can use us under any circumstances if only we will allow Him the opportunity. It's likely we will not be utilized in the way that we would have chosen. God often waits until we are so drained of our own resources and strength that anything that is accomplished must be attributed solely to Him. We must give Him the glory, and as we share how He worked through our weaknesses, we encourage those around us who are skeptical about how God will be able to use them. Talking to the woman at the well was hardly a glamourous assignment, but God does not choose to work in ways that serve our own self.

Lord, I can be sure that I won't ever have a bungy jumping ministry, but You will work out Your plan for my life in Your timing and with Your strength. Help me be patient. ~Lisa Copen

Must I Give Thanks?

"In everything give thanks. For this is the will of God in Christ Jesus concerning you," (1 Thessalonians 5:18).

When I was first diagnosed with an illness, I was told, "You're so lucky you got this illness at such a young age when there is so much research going on." And "You should be thankful. God is going to use it to do incredible things." Although this may be true, "Give thanks!" is not something to tell one who feels her life crumbling out from under her.

1 Thessalonians 5:18 states, "In everything give thanks. For this is the will of God in Christ Jesus concerning you." Sometimes it can feel like God is mocking us when we read that. Does He really expect us to give thanks? Perhaps, God means that only *through* Him will we be able to still find something in which to give thanks, even in the worst of circumstances. God will *enable* us to be thankful in our circumstances; thus, we will become better disciples.

In Philip Yancey's book *Where is God When it Hurts,* he states, "Rejoicing in suffering does not mean Christians should act happy about tragedy and pain when they feel like crying. Rather, the Bible aims the spotlight on the end result, the productive use God can make of suffering in our lives."[8]

I like that better. God says *in* everything, not *for* everything, give thanks. Tears are okay. Eventually, I will grow tired of tear-stained cheeks, however, and focus on what God can do within my circumstances. It's my choice. C. S. Lewis wrote, "Every time you make a choice, you are turning the central part of you, the part that chooses, into something a little different from what it was before."[9] Only through faith am I able to stand up to a tragedy and let it be a blessing.

Lord, only through my relationship with You can I make the lemonade, rather than just suck on the lemons, that life has granted.

~Lisa Copen

Jesus Understands

"There some people brought to Him a man who was deaf and could hardly talk, and they begged Him to place His hand on the man. After He took him aside, away from the crowd, Jesus put His fingers into the man's ears…He looked up to heaven and with a deep sigh said to him, 'Ephphatha!' [Be opened]," (Mark 7:32-34).

I love this story in the Gospel of Mark because we are shown how Jesus ministers to us in such a personal way, with deep compassion toward us when we are hurting. In this event, after Jesus had taken the deaf and dumb man away from the crowd, as He was ministering to the man, it says that He sighed.

God sighed! One can only speculate what He was sighing about, but I believe that our Lord was overwhelmed with the suffering that humanity has to endure. In another gospel, it says that Jesus wept as He was at the scene of a family who was grieving the death of a loved one, (John 11:35). Imagine that! God cried because He empathized so deeply with our grief.

Pain, sickness, death—our Lord Jesus encountered all of these continuously while He was here on earth. We must remember that Jesus empathizes with us in our suffering. He paid the price for it, through His death and separation from God for three days. When my body is filled by pain, I become afraid, but I can go to Him and share my deepest feelings; He will not belittle me or make me feel ashamed of the fears. He won't lecture me or dismiss me. "[Jesus] was despised and rejected by men, a man of sorrows, and familiar with suffering," (Isaiah 53:3). Go to Jesus and share your deepest feelings and fears with Him.

Lord, You understand perfectly what I am experiencing. I want to be transparent with You, so draw me close to Your loving heart. Whisper words of encouragement, hope, and love to my needy spirit.

~Virginia Ganskie

Why Am I Not Healed?

"'Rabbi, who sinned, this man or his parents, that he was born blind?' 'Neither this man nor his parents sinned,' said Jesus, 'but this happened so that the work of God might be displayed in his life,'" (John 9:2,3).

The other day I was talking with a friend, and she asked me how I was feeling. Then she said, "I can't imagine why God hasn't healed you. Maybe you aren't getting the message!" I know that I am hardly the first person to be told these words, and yet they still sting. At one time, I too wondered *What have I done to deserve this? I've led a decent life, so why isn't God healing me?* As time has passed, however, I have surrendered to God the need to be physically healed. I trust He knows what is best for me, and that is all the answer that I need. My friend is not alone in wondering if I perhaps did something to bring this misfortune on myself. Jesus' own disciples asked the same thing when they met a man who was blind from birth. "Rabbi, who sinned, this man or his parents, that he was born blind?" they asked, (John 9:2).

This isn't an easy concept to grasp. Our world believes that success will be rewarded and tragedies are the consequence of bad behavior and poor choices. How can God be glorified by something which our world views as a bad fortune? A wise author who lived in London in the 1600's once wrote, "Sometimes God delays the answer to our prayer in final form, until we have time to build up the strength, accumulate the knowledge, or, fashion the character, that would make it possible for Him to say yes to what we ask," (Samuel Pepys).[10] God's ways are not our ways and His thoughts are not our thoughts. It would be hopeless to try to "figure out God."

God, as Your Son approached His death, He had every reason to question Your reasons, but He simply said, "Father, into Your hands I commit My spirit," (Luke 23:46). Give me this kind of trust.

~Lisa Copen

Deep Waters

"When you pass through the waters, I will be with you; and when you pass through the rivers, they will not sweep over you," (Isaiah 43:2).

With unseeing eyes, I flipped through the pages of a magazine. Tossing the magazine on the table, I glanced around the clinic's waiting room. Were all these people as anxious and fidgety as I? New symptoms drove me to this doctor's office. Severe muscle spasms in my neck and shoulders now joined my array of bodily complaints.

Although painful, these muscular warning signs did not prepare me for the doctor's words, "You have fibromyalgia." Relief that I now had a name for my symptoms crashed against the heavy dread of coping with a second chronic disease. Already overwhelmed with physical maladies, this new disease threatened to drown me.

In Isaiah 43:2, God does not promise to be with us *if* we face difficulties; He promises His presence *when* we encounter troubled waters. Hard times are inevitable in this life, but God is right there in the surging river with us. In addition, God does not leave us floundering in the water. In the introduction to her book *Lord of My Rocking Boat,* Carole Mayhall states, "God says 'through the waters' which means there is the other side."[11] Not only do we have God's promise of His presence; God will also deliver us to the "other side" of our difficulties.

In the years since I was diagnosed with fibromyalgia, God has brought me through many rivers of flare-ups and infections. If I cling to Him, I will not drown, no matter how rough the current.

Lord, thank You that You are with me in the midst of life's troubled waters. Help me trust You to bring me safely to the other side.

~Judy Gann

When Life Is Bittersweet

"So then, those who suffer according to God's will should commit themselves to their faithful Creator and continue to do good," (1 Peter 4:19).

It was to be an event of a lifetime. Ron Karnaugh, the world's highest ranked swimmer in the two-hundred individual medley, was competing in the 1992 Summer Olympics in Barcelona. Ron's proud 61-year-old father, Peter, climbed the steps of the stadium to take a photograph of his son. He never made it to the top. He suffered a fatal heart attack. Despite the tragedy, Ron decided to compete in the Barcelona Games and ultimately finished sixth in the two-hundred individual medley final. Later, following his mother's battle with throat cancer, he decided to go to medical school to become a physician.

God doesn't waste our suffering. Revelation 2:10 warns us, "Do not be afraid of what you are about to suffer." 1 Peter 4:12 prepares us with the words, "Dear friends, do not be surprised at the painful trial you are suffering, as though something strange were happening to you." We will have days of joy and days of passion. We will also have days of suffering. There will also be moments that are bittersweet, as we watch our joys and sufferings intersect, expressing an emotion in our soul that words will never be able to explain.

I had a good "life plan," but God's intervention destroyed those plans rather than blessed them. We must embrace God's plans. You are exactly where He wants you to be today, and not a moment is being wasted. He's completing the circle to glorify Him in a way we never planned for or expected.

Lord, I grasp firmly onto Your hand to guide me through these troubling and confusing times. I still live here on earth, where things are less than perfect, but Your love is perfectly designed to meet my every need. *~Lisa Copen*

What Really Matters

"Beloved, I pray that you may prosper in all things and be in health, just as your soul prospers," (1 John 1:2).

Those of us coping with chronic illness may feel dismayed when we first read this verse of scripture. Our thought is, "Health sounds pretty good to me!" However, I recently read something that made me perceive this scripture differently. What kind of health is most important: physical health or spiritual health?

The following story reminded me that spiritual health is most significant. William Sangster, British Methodist leader during World War II, contracted a disease that paralyzed his body and vocal cords. On the Easter before he died, he scribbled this note: "How terrible to wake up on Easter and have no voice to shout, 'He is Risen!' Far worse, to have a voice and not want to shout."

We cannot always have the physical health we desire. We say, "My eyes fail, looking for Your promise, [Lord]; I say, 'When will You comfort me?'" (Psalm 119:82). We can, however, control our spiritual health, and that's truly what is important. God is often nearer to us in sickness than when we have good physical health, due to our relationship with Him. When we draw near to God, He draws near to us.

Joni Eareckson Tada wrote, "Whatever suffering you are going through this minute, your reaction to it affects the eternity you will enjoy. Heaven will be more heavenly to the degree that you have followed Christ on earth."[12] My friend, we can truly know the joy of the Lord even while we are coping with chronic pain and illness.

Lord, be near as I meet You in prayer; I believe in Your Word. This will bring me the health that matters, and I will know peace, even in the pain. Heaven will be even sweeter since I have suffered.

~Patricia Armstrong

I'm Stressed Out, Lord

"Trust in Him at all times, O people; pour out your hearts to Him, for God is our Refuge," (Psalm 62:8).

It is obvious that stress can make our illnesses react negatively; yet when people tell me this, I want to reply, "If I wasn't ill, I wouldn't be stressed!" It's a catch-22 situation.

My chiropractor says he would rather treat someone after a fall than someone dealing with ongoing stress. A person who falls will heal faster. When I was particularly stressed out, he told me I was "internalizing" and I needed to find a stress outlet. He shared how some of his patients read, some walked, some prayed.

I pray! But as I mulled over his words, I realized I pray, sing, walk, and praise. . . unless I get extremely overwhelmed. Then I tend to clam up and hold everything inside. It is as if I am trying to be tough and strong, even for God.

How unnecessary. I don't need to pretend for Him. God is our refuge. Prayer is His prescribed stress outlet for us. Yes, He already knows all that is occurring in our lives and how we feel about it, but He wants to hear it from us. The Bible says we are to pour out our hearts to Him. Pour it all out! Be honest. Get it out there. The Lord God wants to hear your unpolished cries. He wants to hear your real heart. He can take the questions. He can take the anger. He will comfort the hurt. His greatest desire is authentic intimacy.

But we have to go to Him. He waits for us with arms open wide. He wants us to give Him all our pressures, stress, and worry. "Cast all your anxiety on Him because He cares for you," (I Peter 5:7). We can relax and let God take over.

Lord God Almighty, You care for me and can handle anything and everything that comes my way. What sweet relief. ~*Erica Faraone*

Change My Heart

"Many are the plans in a man's heart, but it is the Lord's purpose that prevails," (Proverbs 19:21).

Many times have I prayed, asking God to take away my pain or even the side effects of the medications. Many times have I wished that I could go back in time fifteen years and prevent my accident. During the first years following, I asked God to heal me. I wanted my old life back, the things I had been able to do before, the enjoyment of life I had always known.

I grew up in a Christian family and was active in my local church; Most of my social life revolved around my church activities and church friends. I believed that God had a plan for my life. I felt His guidance in making leadership decisions in my service for Him.

After the accident, as time wore on, it seemed that God was telling me that, although He was able to take away my pain, He was not going to. I understood Job's thoughts, "My days have passed, my plans are shattered, and so are the desires of my heart," (Job 17:11). I realized I was now going to have to learn to live with chronic pain from the soft tissue damage to my neck and back and the peripheral problems. It's hard to not let pain rule one's life. Sometimes it is so severe that pain is all one can think about. It is no surprise we ask God to change our circumstances, but His desire is for us to ask Him for the grace and strength to live through them. Our hearts need to be focused on God to be able to accept His answer.

The Reverend Dr. Dale Turner says, "Dreams are renewable. No matter what our age or condition, there are still untapped possibilities within us and new beauty waiting to be born."

Knowing that You, God, daily strive to help me change my heart, my attitude, and help me reach my dreams, to serve You, keeps me going regardless of the circumstances I face.

~Fiona Burrows

Who Was I Back Then?

"Do not say, 'Why were the old days better than these?' For it is not wise to ask such questions," (Ecclesiastes 7:10).

I was determined to clean out my clothes closet before the sun set on that day. Hangers no longer hung on the bar, but rather dangled from other hangers. The overflowing clothes needed to be sorted. It was a job I was not eager to tackle.

As I neared the back of the closet, cleaning became less of a physical undertaking and more of an emotional journey. Scarves drooped from the scarf rack, limp with dust. Bright-colored belts, adorned with jewels and stones, hung without the luster they had once shown. Piles of shoes that had long since been abadandoned were heaped in the corner, and fun hats lined the top shelf, thick with dust. *Who was this woman?* I asked myself. Gazing at the items I had once worn with ease, I knew the answer. She was me—before illness.

When rheumatoid arthritis took possession of my body, the scarves became burdensome, as I searched for any semblance of comfort. The shoes stopped fitting onto my feet, and heels became impossible to stand in. For a time, I had no place to wear my fancy clothes, and then, as steroids increased my weight, the clothes just no longer fit.

I've heard the saying, "Dig yourself a pit and you're likely to fall into it." Digging through my closet could have been a pit of pity, yet I realized this, had a good cry, grieved my losses, and then moved on. In some ways, the old days were better than these. At twenty-something, I felt confident with my body; after years of struggling with my weight as a child, I was finally a size six and enjoying that freedom. Now I am, I'll admit, larger than a six, but I know God more intimately.

I know what is important in this lifetime. I have a different kind of confidence and in it the joy in knowing You, Lord, and believing You are all I need. Hats not required. ~Lisa Copen

What Do You Want From Me?

"He has showed you, O man, what is good. And what does the Lord require of you? To act justly and to love mercy and to walk humbly with your God," (Micah 6:8).

I often ask God, "What do You want from me?" I am very confused about what the Lord wants from my life. I find myself almost resentful or discouraged when I think about how lacking I am physically, spiritually, and emotionally. At times, my faults and weaknesses seem to glare at me, becoming larger and more intense, as if they were zooming in to overtake me. During these times, I feel overwhelmed, like a useless being in God's eyes.

Yet, as I read this verse in Micah, I am comforted by what it says. I am reminded that God requires the same of each of His children. The Lord does not ask more of us than we can carry out. I see in this verse that we should act justly, which is no easy task when struggling against the selfish pulls of the flesh, yet we have God's power to do it. Secondly, we are to love mercy. Loving mercy means showing mercy to others the way you have been shown mercy from the Lord. This can seem to be another monstrous task at times. Our human nature instinctively judges, blames, or faults others for their predicament, rather than shows compassion. Our human character wants someone to blame for the hurts, fears, and trials. We are called to endure.

Lastly, we are to walk humbly with God. We must look to God to provide our every need, as little children who rely solely on the providence of their parents, never doubting, but trusting them. Walking humbly means daily submitting to God's will in our lives. Walking humbly means admitting our needs, faults and mistakes mistakes and asking God to give us strength to overcome our weaknesses.

May I walk humbly with You, God, today, acting justly and showing compassion and mercy to all I encounter. *~Tina Nahid*

It's So Hard To Ask For Help

"Surely God is my help; the Lord is the one who sustains me," (Psalm 54:4).

In the past, I could grab a ladder, hammer, and nail and have a picture on the wall in less than five minutes. Now, I have to ask my husband for help, and an hour later, he is still measuring, leveling, and consulting. He has also learned that when I say, "when you have time, could you possibly..." it should be interpreted as, "I need you to do this right now."

When the Israelite army was attacked by the Amalekites, (Exodus 17:8-15), Moses stood on top of the hill with the staff of God in his hands. If Moses held his hands up to God, the Israelites would win the battle, but when he let his hands fall, the Amalekites began to win. So, was Moses able to pull through the long hours, holding up his hands? Not without the help of Aaron and Hur. "Aaron and Hur held his hands up—one on one side, one on the other—so that his hands remained steady till sunset," (v. 12).

God's Holy power was flowing through the fingertips of Moses, and yet God still allowed Moses' arms to become tired. Was that so Moses had to accept help? What would have happened if Moses had said, "Don't worry about it, guys. I can handle it. Go on down the hill, and I'll come later when I finish this battle"? God was able to accomplish His purpose through Moses only because Moses accepted the help of others. Although we always have the power of God within us, there are times that He chooses not to release that power unless we humbly accept the help of others, in order to complete His purpose.

Lord, guide me in recognizing that You are always there in times of trouble, but that I have to ask for help and accept it graciously, not apologetically.

~Lisa Copen

Laughter Through Tears

"He who goes out weeping, carrying seeds to sow, will return with songs of joy, carrying shaves with him," (Psalm 126:6).

I remember a line from a movie long ago that said, "The greatest emotion is laughter through tears." A simultaneous burst of sorrow and joy can come at a time when your eyes are red and puffy and suddenly someone says something hysterical and you can't help but laugh. It can come when you are laughing so hard that tears start to form in your eyes, and pretty soon you are doubling over from laughter, yet crying simultaneously. It is such a powerful emotion.

God surely understands the power of tears as He gave Hezekiah fifteen more years of life, when he came to God, weeping bitterly. Hezekiah was ill to the point of death and distraught when the Lord told him, "Put your house in order, because you are going to die; you'll not recover," (Isaiah 38:1). After Hezekiah's tears and plea, God told Isaiah, "Go and tell Hezekiah, 'This is what the Lord, the God of your father David, says: I have heard your prayer and seen your tears; I will add fifteen years to your life,'" (Isaiah 38:3-5).

Tears will bring about joy. Note in Psalm 126:6 the reference to they *will* return with songs of joy, not *might*.

Even Reverend Billy Graham has revealed, "The Christian life is not a constant high. I have my moments of deep discouragement. I have to go to God in prayer with tears in my eyes, and say, 'O God, forgive me,' or 'Help me.'"[13]

Lord, I've been mistaken, believing that by holding in the tears, I am strong. Tears are precious to You, and You count and cherish each salty droplet that stains my cheeks. I have relied too much on my pride and stubbornness, and have robbed You of the opportunity to offer me the comfort that only You can give. Teach me how to cry, Lord.

~Lisa Copen

Learning To Listen

"He who answers before listening – that is his folly and shame. The heart of the discerning acquires knowledge; the ears of the wise seek it out," (Proverbs 18:13,15).

A woman called me and shared her recent diagnosis of a chronic illness. She needed someone who would listen. It was difficult for me to hold back from sharing my own story.

"The heart of the discerning acquires knowledge; the ears of the wise seek it out," says Proverbs 18:15. I was blessed with a friend who had a special gift of drawing one out and then listening intently to the answers. John went to meet Jesus at the age of 46, but he listened attentively to every person who opened their heart to him, which was nearly everyone who met him. Through a sparkle in his eye and a transfixed gaze on you, John communicated that anything you shared would be treated as the most precious information he had ever heard. He absorbed your answer and treasured it.

Jesus preached as He traveled; He took great time to earnestly listen to the people He met. He held the children and blessed them, but I am sure He also listened to their songs and even held a few of their pet bugs. Jesus asked people questions and listened to their answers. He never assumed to know an answer, such as when He asked the disabled man at the pool, "Would you like to be healed?" Without a doubt, I can say that Jesus kneeled down to this man's level as He spoke to him and then listened for his reply.

It is difficult to abstain from offering people reasuring, "God balm" answers. "God will work it all out" or, "Try to keep the faith." These words come naturally when we don't have answers. It takes effort to sit quietly and let a friend share sorrows, fears, struggles, and pain; but that is friendship, so make the effort. They won't easily forget it.

Lord, help me to be a friend who truly listens. ~Lisa Copen

Daily Divine Protection

"Keep me as the apple of Your eye; hide me in the shadow of Your wings," (Psalm 17:8).

One morning, Abraham, my one-year-old son, was sitting, playing innocently underneath the kitchen table in the sunlight. As I watched him play, I noticed he was going to stand up. I gently and quietly placed my hand underneath the edge of the table, and as I suspected, his head came up and bumped that exact spot. Without his awareness, my hand had cushioned his head and saved him from a "boo-boo."

Just as my hand had been there to protect my child from pain, so is Jesus protecting us. Just as Abraham had no idea of my intervention on his behalf, so we many times never realize how much the Lord God watches over us. We want to hear from God in a profound way. We want God to call to us from a burning bush, as He did Moses. While this communication with the Lord Almighty is very possible and does happen, He also communicates with us through quiet but divine intervention in our everyday lives. "The Lord is faithful, and He will strengthen and protect you from the evil one," (2 Thessalonians 3:3). But yes, sometimes we feel like the psalmist in Psalm 10:1: "Why, O Lord, do You stand far off? Why do You hide Yourself in times of trouble?"

Are you are a child of God? If you believe in His Son, Jesus Christ, have accepted Him as your Savior, and have repented of your past sins, then, my friend, the Lord's protection over you is assured! This doesn't mean that nothing tragic will happen in your life, but it does mean that nothing happens without coming through God's discerning fingers first.

Yearly, daily, hourly, second by second, the Lord's hand of protection is upon us in countless ways.

Lord, help me to realize how much You love me, even when You are quiet in my life.
~Tina Nahid

Can I Laugh Without Guilt?

"Sarah was afraid, so she lied and said, 'I did not laugh.' But He said, 'Yes, you did laugh,'" (Genesis 8:15).

Have you experienced a morning that consisted of getting out of bed, taking a shower, eating breakfast, and still feeling as though you could make some plans for the day? For many, these days are too rare, but when we encounter one, it's exciting... until we begin to feel guilty. Our neighbor questions how we can be in too much pain to work, and yet still be able to pull a few weeds. At the grocery store you run into your child's teacher, who says, "Timmy said you've been ill, but you look great!" Your husband answers the phone and tells your girlfriend you decided to run to a couple of garage sales, the same girlfriend you cancelled lunch plans with two days earlier because you could hardly get out of bed.

We all need more joy, and yet, when it comes we are too afraid to laugh. Like Sarah we say, "I did not laugh. I did not enjoy that too much. I did not have a moment of feeling good, because that will cause skepticism among those around me." When we feel good, we downplay it so that it will even out with all the instances we say we are fine but we aren't.

According to research, children laugh 400 times a day while adults laugh only fifteen times.[14] And a five-year study by the UCLA School of Medicine discovered that laughing boosts the body's natural defenses, enhances pain management and reduces stress-hormone levels. Better yet, one study revealed that a 1-minute "hee-haw" is equal to ten minutes on a rowing machine—and it's more fun.[15] Throw caution to the wind. Laugh! Sarah said, "God has brought me laughter, and everyone who hears about this will laugh with me," (Genesis 21:6). You don't owe anyone an explanation. Say, "Isn't it incredible? I can hardly believe that I am out and about like this. I decided to enjoy it while I could!"

Lord, help me invite everyone to laugh with me. ~Lisa Copen

Knowing Where You're Needed

"The King will reply, 'I tell you the truth, whatever you did for one of the least of these brothers of mine, you did for Me,'" (Matthew 25:40).

Our neighbor passed away of cancer. Before his passing, unbeknownst to us, another neighbor had witnessed to him. "What?" I exclaimed when my husband told me. We didn't even know our newest neighbors were believers.

I watched the cars come and go across the street for a few days; as it grew quieter, I made some brownies, and my husband and I walked over with them. His wife appeared at the door and invited us in and told us for the next forty-five minutes how the Lord had blessed them. She cried and shared how it was the hardest thing she had ever gone through; she was going to just take one day at a time.

"I feel so awful," I explained. "We didn't know. Here I sit across the street with a chronic illness ministry. . . and you and your husband are going through this!" His immaculate lawn had turned brown this winter. I should have realized. I should have knocked on the door—just because—and waited to see if they shared anything they were going through.

Yes, we are each in pain. Daily, we deal with so much, but it could be so much harder. While we wait for people to just "understand" our predicament of living with illness, others, in their last days, wait for their loved ones to come and simply say their goodbyes. Illness gives us compassion and understanding, but we must be willing to let God use us. I got wrapped up in "stuff" and missed a blessed opportunity outside my front door.

Lord, help me listen more clearly for Your voice so You can lead me back across the street when I am needed. *~Lisa Copen*

Being Me

"Commit to the Lord whatever you do, and your plans will succeed. The Lord works out everything for His own ends," (Proverbs 16:3,4).

As a child, I found growing up very difficult. I liked to play by myself; tea parties were attended by my dolls and teddy bears. I was shy and withdrawn. As I grew, many people wounded me with malicious comments. It hurt me to the core of my soul, and I pledged to God that someday my life would mean something; one day, people would look at me with honor and respect.

Isn't that what we all want—to be needed and appreciated for who we are? It can feel like we are Hester Prynne in *The Scarlet Letter*, wearing the words "Chronic Illness" across our clothes. Beloved, living with chronic illness and pain does not define us. Yes, it is a part of who we are, but it does not define our hopes or the dreams we can long for.

We are all limited beings, not just because of our ailments, but because we are human. We are imperfect beings, struggling due to our medical problems, and longing for a life we once knew. Yet, we don't understand that there may be new paths for us to reach for. Many of us are wonderful with our hands and may choose to crochet blankets for neonatal babies in the hospital. Some may want to teach a young child how to fish or cook. Write an autobiography about your life as a child or how you have managed to cope each day with your conditions.

Most importantly, know this: God loves you. He knows the trials you face, for He experienced them Himself in the human form of Jesus, His Son. Jesus felt our fears and trials, and He feels yours too.

Let me not become weary in doing good, for at the proper time I will reap a harvest if I do not give up, (Galatians 6:9). *~Kay DeCarlo*

Recognizing Evil

"There is no fear in love. But perfect love drives out fear, because fear has to do with punishment. The one who fears is not made perfect in love," (1 John 4:18).

The sun is shining through the blinds, and my eyes peek from under the sheets, basking in the relaxation of the morning. I notice my body is still and not agitated. There is no pain. In fact, I feel pretty well. I slide out of bed. . . still no pain. What a perfect morning! Have you ever felt this way? For someone with a chronic condition, mornings like this are precious. Sometimes, however, just as we are glowing from within, an insidious voice invades our thoughts, *"Yeah, you feel good now, but when is it going to end? This won't last. You know that you will be in pain later."*

My friend, that voice is not the voice of our Lord Jesus, and it's not even your voice. That voice is from the pit and from the snake who wants you with him. You see, Satan knows that, although the Lord's perfect love covers you completely for eternity, he can try to make you become fearful and doubt God's promises. If he can make your patience with God wear thin by using your illness, as he did with Job, he will. We must remember 1 John 4:18: "There is no fear in love. But perfect love drives out fear, because fear has to do with punishment. The one who fears is not made perfect in love."

Oswald Chambers says, "We all know people who have been made much meaner, more irritable, and more intolerable to live with by suffering; it is not right to say that all suffering perfects. It only perfects one type of person… the one who accepts the call of God in Christ Jesus."[16]

Lord, teach me to recognize evil and how it can manipulate my thoughts. Let me be steadfast in You with trust, hope, and faith in the plans You have for my life so that I can accept Your call and be made perfect in Your timing. *~Tina Nahid*

I Don't Want To Just Survive

"Being confident of this, that He who began a good work in you will carry it on to completion until the day of Christ Jesus," (Philippians 1:6).

The front of a greeting card, attributed to poet Maya Angelou, reads, "Surviving is important. Thriving is elegant."[17] I bought a package of the cards, and then I framed one for my desk. Surviving is admirable, and every day I live in some state of survival. However, I don't want to feel like my life is a stretching exercise, consistently trying to just accomplish the basics. I want to live! I want to have some fun! I want to be able to serve the Lord in mighty ways. Don't I need a healthy body to do this?

No. In my opinion, surviving is what we do each day. Thriving is the attitude we must have while surviving! Despite the wonderful plans I had for my healthy life, the Lord had other plans, and they included illness. Each day, the Lord's plans continue to include illness. Today, they do not include healing. They do not include remission. They do not even include pain-free moments. The Lord's plans, however, do include thriving. They include elegance, because we are living the exact life that God wants us to live, a life we never would have discovered without the thorn of the illness.

A seventy-seven-year-old woman emailed me recently. "I am legally blind and have peripheral neuropathy and a deteriorating spine. My best friend is eighty-seven years old, and helps me with our church's homebound ministry. Discussing our ailments, she said, 'Well, Novie, as long as God has something for us to do, these old bodies will last!' It encouraged me; I feel like Paul and would rather go home to be with Jesus, but I am willing to do whatever I can for Him while He leaves me here!"

Yes, surviving is important, thriving is elegant. With You, Lord, I can reach for elegance each day. *~Lisa Copen*

Where Are My Friends?

"My friends and companions avoid me because of my wounds. My neighbors stay far away," (Psalm 38:11).

I stopped by the church office and discovered that one of the staff members had caught the flu. Her spouse was there and said how wonderfully the church had responded to the needs of their family. "We've received at least one meal every day for over a week!" he said. "People have been doing our ironing and cleaning the house. It almost makes it worth getting sick!" (Would she agree?)

I was pleased to hear how responsive the church had been to the family's needs, and yet I was also discouraged. What about all of the chronically ill people that attend the church? How often have they received a meal, had their house cleaned, or even received a card that said, "I am thinking of you"? Unfortunately, people don't really understand how to respond to those with chronic illness. They are hesitant to bring meals until a person is back on her feet, because it is likely that her condition may never improve. The needs of the chronically ill vary, depending on the disease, its progression, the person's age, and even the weather. It's hard to offer comfort when one doesn't know what to offer. I've heard the saying, "Bitterness is like a snowball. It eventually leads to an avalanche." But Samuel Johnson reminds us, "Kindness is in our power, even when fondness is not."[18]

We often feel lonely when people don't respond to *our* pain with cards, child-care, meals, and even ironing. We may even believe that no one cares. What we must remember is that it is very likely people do care, they just don't understand *how* to show us that they care.

Lord, wounds make people uncomfortable, and some may turn away, but many will not. Help me take the time to reach out to those people who care for me and not let pride stand in my way of asking for help when I am in need. ~*Lisa Copen*

I Have No Secrets From God

"All my longings lie open before You, O Lord; my sighing is not hidden from You," (Psalm 38:9).

I don't get angry at God very often. I have accepted my circumstances, dealt with the emotions, and have tried to move on, having a life of joy and not bitterness. I do, however, have moments of sheer annoyance with God. When the side effects pile on top of each other, when doctors say, "We just don't know what else to do for you," when the car won't start and the checking account is overdrawn, I tend to express these moments of annoyance without apology. *Lo-r-d! I am doing the best I can here! Can't You work with me a bit? What more do You want from me?*

I am not condoning my childish whining, but I do think that, ironically, God understands my honesty. I believe that He would rather have me express to Him the emotions that I am feeling, than avoid conversation with Him altogether. "All my longings lie open before You, O Lord; my sighing is not hidden from You," says David in Psalm 38:9. *All* my longings lie open before God, not just the appropriate, unselfish ones.

"The longer I live, the more convinced I become that life is ten percent what happens to us and ninety percent how we respond to it," says Chuck Swindoll. "Attitude keeps me going or cripples my progress. It alone fuels my fire or assaults my hope. When my attitudes are right, there's no barrier too high, no valley too deep, no dream too extreme, no challenge too great for me."[19]

Lord, I feel exasperated with trying to figure You out sometimes. You've heard my sighings, and You understand that I don't understand all that Your plan encompasses for me. I trust that You will offer comfort and reassurance. You want me to come and converse my feelings with You. Thank goodness Your greatest desire is an authentic relationship, where I can be real!

~Lisa Copen

Walking With Jesus

"Scorn has broken my heart and has left me helpless; I looked for sympathy, but there was none, for comforters, but I found none," (Psalm 69:20).

I frequently go on walks with friends, but the exercise is physically and emotionally challenging. I am conscious that I am slowing everyone else down. I simply cannot keep up as they stride by me like the hare dashing off to the finish line. They playfully hurry me along, making me more frustrated. I am the tortoise moseying along, the slowpoke. Living with chronic illness in a fast-paced world is uncomfortable. It takes all of my effort just to get out of bed while my mind's eagerness battles with its slow body.

Rejection overcomes me as the distance between myself and the others grow. Heartbroken, I slow my pace. I keep my gaze focused, however, passing a street lamp, then a tree. I smell the scent of flowers. I smile at the mailbox painted white with black polka dots. As I turn the corner, I see everyone ahead, calling out and waving to me. I am hurt; I am in last place.

Then warmth sweeps beside me. Like a father extending his hand out to his child, Jesus is smiling His greatest smile of comfort. I take hold of His hand. My Jesus waits for me. He is my goal; I focus solely on Him. I continue every step of my walk with Him. I can choose to be calm. It is an admirable option.

Each landmark in our lives is cause for celebration. Living with chronic illness or pain does not need to be isolating. We do not have to keep up with others when we can walk with Jesus. Holding hands with Jesus, we will reach the finish line.

Others do not understand this pace of life I am living, Lord. Heavenly Father, You promise to never leave me behind. You are always right beside me. Thank You. ~*Ellie O'Steen*

God Understands Frustration

"My dear brothers, take note of this: Everyone should be quick to listen, slow to speak and slow to become angry, for man's anger does not bring about the righteous life that God desires," (James 1:19,20).

Anger and frustration are two things I constantly have to deal with while coping with chronic illness. I remember the many ways God has blessed and helped me. I have seen many times how God's fingerprints are upon situations that could have gone very badly but didn't. Still, when I am taking another "hit" with my affliction, the anger and frustration begin to rise like the temperature on a scorching summer day.

Sometimes, the anger is about the worsening of my condition; other times, it is over how I am being limited by my condition. There are instances when a careless or callous word about my condition can cause my temperature to boil and pour over into frustration. "Don't rush right into your anger," writes Novotni and Petersen, authors of *Angry with God*. "The events or perceptions that made you angry have probably sparked a process that has led you through disappointment, feelings of betrayal and abandonment, and a sense of being alone, which may bring sadness, cynicism, and weariness. Don't deny what you feel just because it is not an emotion that others approve of. Claim your feelings."[20]

God is the only one who can bring me peace in these times. All the tranquilizers and pain pills in the world cannot help me keep my perspective and find peace like God can.

He must be the first one we call upon when things are going badly. We cannot afford to wait until we boil over with frustration.

Thank You, God, for being there with me in my good times and my bad times and for understanding my human emotions.

~Karlton Douglas

Remembering To Mourn

"Blessed are those who mourn, for they will be comforted," (Matthew 5:4).

It has become increasingly difficult to hold a fork. As my hand becomes stiff and the joints swell, I struggle to balance the food and get it to my mouth before it falls off the fork. I feel clumsy, embarrassed, and ungraceful. I eat with my left hand, but with little improvement. I've tried hard to avoid the emotions this causes; yet, I am gradually seeing more abilities progress from being difficult to impossible. I try not to face the reality that the degeneration will never stop.

Mourning is a natural part of living with a chronic illness. Each time I believe I have adapted to the changes, I am required to make more adjustments. We've heard how it is healthy to mourn our losses and take time to grieve, but it is also a spiritual blessing. Matthew 5:4 says, "Blessed are those who mourn, for they will be comforted." Through God's grace I can be comforted. If I choose to avoid my feelings and deny my losses, I will miss out on God's blessings and His comfort. It's one thing I can't afford to lose.

It is never easy to admit that things are changing. I long to relive the days when I could get up, shower, dress, and start the day with a burst of energy. Those days are gone; yet I feel embraced by the Lord's promises, which He will fulfill. When I shower and go back to bed, if I listen closely, I can hear God's voice reassuring me that His love will never fail. Although our lives may be filled with losses, we will never lose our Father's love. God has not abandoned us. Of this I am sure! I just needed to let go of my firm grasp on my dreams and shift my focus to His dreams for me so I don't miss His ultimate plan.

Looking back, God, I realize You were gracious enough to intertwine my dreams and Your plans together. You always knew how I would serve You. *~Lisa Copen*

We Are Beautiful To Him

"Your beauty should come from the inner self, the unfading beauty of a gentle and quiet spirit, which is of great worth in God's sight," (1 Peter 3:4).

If I stopped today in front of the mirror, the image I would see before me could be quite frightful. I would see an aging and sickly body, a face filled with pain and sorrow, years of distress, and grief that has taken its toll on my outer appearance. I can masquerade my outer appearance, make it appear more lively and attractive, but I am only hiding the evidence. Inside, my heart still knows the pain and misery.

Depression and illness can make us see "bad" when it isn't even there. We may envision all the sin in our lives, past and present, as scars too frightful to look upon. We may think of ourselves in negative terms and assume that the world, and even God, would be repulsed by our appearance.

Have you heard the expression, "Beauty is not skin deep?" It is hard to grasp this concept if we are judging ourselves too harshly. We tend to let our low self-esteem fill us with doubts and negativity; it leaves us feeling alone and painfully abandoned. Take heart, dear loved one! The Lord God reminds us in 1 Peter 3:4 that He looks at the inner beauty. God created you in His image. You are beautifully fashioned after the image of the Lord. Your heart portrays the beauty of your persona. You are not an outcast. You are not alone.

We are all scarred from the traumas of life. Don't let low self-esteem or depression fill you with emptiness and sorrow. You are a wonderful and beautiful individual, molded and fashioned by the Great Potter and Creator. The Lord sees your inner beauty, and God loves you!

You know my pain, Lord, and You promise to carry me through this trial if I turn to You. There is nothing You cannot forgive, so I cling to Your forgiveness and trust You. ~*Deborah Farmer*

A Friend's Fight Is Over

"I have fought the good fight, I have finished the race, I have kept the faith," (2 Timothy 4:7,8).

A friend has died. She fought to live for years despite the cancer that wouldn't give up. Finally, God took her home. I'm so angry, and I just want to yell at God, *How can You do this? How can You call yourself merciful by taking this incredible woman, mother, and wife? Where is the justice?*

Paul wrote, "I have fought the good fight, I have finished the race, I have kept the faith," (2 Timothy 4:7,8). How did Paul know that he had finished the race? Paul did not have an easy life. He was tired, both physically and emotionally. Perhaps he was ready. But my friend was not. She still had young children and had recently been blessed with her first grandchild. She was still fighting and still in the race.

It is moments like this I can hardly begin to understand God's ways. I make a mental note to add another question to my list of when-I-get-to-heaven-answers. I cling to the fact that I know that God has designed a course for each of our lives. It is not the length of life, it's the depth and strength with which one lived. It's the faith that one had and the spirit of God that they shared with those around them. I hope when my time comes, I will be able to say, "I have run a good race. I am ready." I seriously doubt I will have this attitude, however. I think I will still be hanging on, asking God to let me run just one more mile. Situations like my friend's passing throw me back into the reality that life is short and nothing can be taken for granted. Life is a gift. I have so much life I want to experience. I had better get busy and make every moment count.

"Show me, O Lord, my life's end and the number of my days; let me know how fleeting is my life. You have made my days a mere handbreadth; the span of my years is as nothing before You. Each man's life is but a breath," (Psalm 39:4,5). *~Lisa Copen*

Make God Your Strength And Shield

"The Lord is my strength and my shield; my heart trusts in Him and I am helped," (Psalm 28:7).

As I was reading in Psalms, this verse jumped out and stayed with me. "My heart trusts in Him and I am helped." We will be helped when we learn to let go and trust that God has everything—past, present, and future—under control. Nothing in our life has, or will, take the Lord by surprise. That means He has allowed the exact circumstances in which we now find ourselves.

This knowledge may make us angry at first. *If He knew how much pain I'd be in, why did He allow this illness?* To find peace on this point, we have to trust His love. We have to choose to believe that He desires and enacts that which will be the very best for our lives. Often, we find better health, inside and out, from surrender alone.

"A heart at peace gives life to the body, but envy rots the bones," (Proverbs 14:30). We will find a better frame of mind when we have a heart at peace. However, if we envy others, even of their health, our outlook will quickly darken; it seems our body follows the lead of our heart and mind when it comes to attitude.

This is one of the reasons we need to keep our mind on the Lord. "You will keep in perfect peace him whose mind is steadfast, because he trusts in you," (Isaac 26:3). If we really trust the Lord God, our minds will be unwavering, and we will be at peace. We will find help, comfort, and rest in His love and His perfect ways.

Lord, I will relax and trust You—with my circumstances, my illness, my pain, my fatigue, my bills, my body, and my very life. Let me find my help in trusting in Your great plan for my life.

~Erica Faraone

The View I Didn't Want

"They went up on the roof and lowered him on his mat through the tiles into the middle of the crowd. . ." (Luke 5:19).

As I reflect on this verse, I often wonder, did the man ask his friends to help him go to see Jesus? Was he embarrassed about the hole they carved to lower him down? Was he one who didn't like to call attention to his disabilities? It's easy to see the loving-kindness of his friends, who went so far out of their way to get him near the healing salve of the Lord, and yet, was it difficult for the man to accept their help? Did people stare and ask one another, "Do you think he's really that bad? Did he just not want to wait in line to get inside?"

I won't forget my first experience of riding in a wheelchair. My family was visiting from out of state, and we had planned to go to Disneyland. I knew that I could not walk around the park, and so I agreed to use the wheelchair. By the time we got there, it was raining, but we bought Mickey umbrellas and capes and decided to have fun anyway. I have to admit, the rain didn't bother me. . . but the wheelchair did.

I felt embarrassed as people with looks of suspicion watched me. Kids kicked my legs and shoved the chair to get by, as if I was not human. Their parents watched without comment. I couldn't participate in the small talk. I was mad that I had to be in the ugly chair and that my family had chosen an outing in which I was forced to use it. Trying to help, they would push me right up to the restroom door, not realizing I needed to walk; other times, I was forgotten, and I had to get up and push the chair to catch up with them. It was a learning experience for us all, but more so, a grieving experience. I was too frustrated to make *them* comfortable. My dad bit back tears. My mom tried to make us have fun. My husband tried to protect me, and figure out how to comfort me.

Lord, let me always remember to listen to those who find themselves with a view they didn't want. ~Lisa Copen

Is God Really On My Side?

"'Do not be terrified; do not be afraid of them. The Lord your God, Who is going before you, will fight for you, as He did for you in Egypt, before your eyes, and in the desert. There you saw how the Lord your God carried you, as a father carries his son, all the way you went until you reached this place," (Deuteronomy 1:29-31).

Prior to entering the Promised Land, Moses spoke to the Israelites, who were upset. "You grumbled in your tents and said, 'The Lord hates us; so He brought us out of Egypt to deliver us into the hands of the Amorites to destroy us,'" (Deuteronomy 1:27). Have you ever cried out, *God, why do you hate me? Why are you trying to destroy me?* Do you feel helpless, as if you were up against a city of giants? Perhaps you feel as if you are in a losing battle after wandering in the desert. When I realize I can't fight this battle alone, I allow God to carry me. I have a choice, as did the Israelites: I can surrender to despair and defeat, or surrender to God, letting Him fight for me. I've done both; the latter is far more rewarding!

I don't fully comprehend why God allows us to suffer to the point of excruciating pain, but I know this: God does not hate you! He loved you enough to die for you. The Scriptures bring me such consolation. When I begin to feel punished, I read the words of the Psalmist, David or Job, or the weeping prophet who wrote the Book on Lamenting! I know it can sure feel like God's wrath when I'm in agony; yet, I find the very same emotions put into words by these men of God. David was "a man after God's own heart"; Job was "blameless and upright"; and God said "there [was] no one on earth like Him." What hope this brings to my soul! You see, I know how the story ends for all these men of faith, and it encourages me. I am not alone.

"I called on Your name, O Lord, from the depths of the pit. You heard my plea: 'Do not close Your ears to my cry for relief.' You came near when I called You, and You said, 'Do not fear,'" (Lamentations 3:55-57).

~Lori Mortensen

I Long For Real Sleep

"I will lie down and sleep in peace, for You alone, O Lord, make me dwell in safety," (Psalm 4:8).

The reception desk at my doctor's office has a plaque that says, "Don't take your worries to bed. Give them to God. He's up all night anyway!" How I long for some sleep. My body craves peace, rest, and deep sleep. No matter how much time I spend in bed, however, I never seem to feel renewed. One of the most difficult changes to adjust to is the constant fatigue that accompanies chronic illness. Just doing the dishes brings about an exhaustion I have never experienced.

"Exhaust" is from the Latin root word which means "to draw out." I feel used up. It scares me to think that I may never know the level of energy I once possessed. My eyes crave darkness and stillness; my body longs for the warm comforts of my grandmother's quilt. Perhaps it is hardest to accept that, even if these longings were fulfilled, I would still awake wishing for more sleep, never feeling refilled. I want to fall asleep and awake feeling like I did "before illness."

Fortunately, God understands this desire for sleep and renewal. The Psalmist David says, "I will lie down and sleep in peace, for You alone, O Lord, make me dwell in safety," (Psalm 4:8). We have a God who will protect us, not only from harm, but from becoming spiritually exhausted and lacking renewal. Victor Hugo reminds us, "Have courage for the great sorrows of life and patience for the small ones. And when you have finished your daily task, go to sleep in peace. God is awake." God is awake, and He understands the craving we have for peaceful sleep. I pray that He will provide that for you tonight.

Despite the pain, the insomnia, and the worries that come late at night, I can find peace in knowing that You will never leave my side, God. You are right there right beside me, wanting to encompass me in Your arms. *~Lisa Copen*

The Waiting Game

"For the Lord comforts His people and will have compassion on His afflicted ones," (Isaiah 49:13).

Waiting. It can be so burdensome at times. Waiting for the pharmacy checkout line to move forward, for doctors' appointments, or for test results. In the midst of all of it, we get lost in the mire.

As new medications are given to help one illness, I am told to stop taking a different one, for it may be giving me another illness. Lab work leads to more tests and the waiting game. "Test results may come in later today," I'm told. "Hopefully, they'll be in tomorrow. Stay tuned," says the nurse. It sounds like a news report. I wait. What next? When will it end?

When anxiety and affliction surround me, I realize how imperative it is that I cling to my faith. We must believe in the promise that God has for us, trusting and believing in the words of Jesus, "I will not leave you as orphans, I will come to you," (John 14:18).

No matter what you are going through, believe Jesus will come to you. He will not abandon you, for you are so loved. He will make a way through it for you to cope. Skeptical? Listen to what God says: "I am the Lord, the God of all mankind. Is anything too hard for Me?" (Jeremiah 32:27). Yes, things can seem hard to comprehend, but God will never let us fall out of His reach.

Sometimes I am so lost, Lord, searching aimlessly for You, not knowing what to do or how to find You. Jesus said, "Come to Me all you who are weary and burdened, and I will give you rest," (Matthew 11:28). I'm here, Lord. I've come. Help me feel You lift the worries and burdens from me. I don't want them anymore.

~Kay DeCarlo

Concentrate

"So we fix our eyes not on what is seen, but on what is unseen; for what is seen is temporary, but what is unseen is eternal," (2 Corinthians 4:18).

I heard an amusing story once about a waitress who was staring at a bottle of orange juice in the restaurant. When a customer asked her what she was doing, she replied, "The label on the bottle says 'concentrate.'" When you suffer from pain, it is hard to concentrate on anything other than the pain. I find that when the pain is forceful, my lack of concentration is more apparent.

When tragedy and pain seem all around us, we tend to fix our eyes on the suffering and sorrow. During these times, when we are in the darkest of days, it seems that pondering on the sadness is inevitable.

The Bible reminds us in 2 Corinthians 4:18 to fix our eyes on what is unseen, not on what we see and "know." The things in this world will perish soon. They are only temporary. The life after this world, however, is forever. What happens when we focus on ourselves? See Job's reaction: "Is my complaint directed to man? Why should I not be impatient? When I think about this, I am terrified; trembling seizes my body," (Job 21:4,6).

Hebrews 12:2 says, "Let us fix our eyes on Jesus."

Even David proclaimed within his suffering, "My eyes are fixed on You, O Sovereign Lord; in You I take refuge. Do not give me over to death," (Psalm 141:8).

Lord, let me concentrate on Your "label" – the Bible. Fix my eyes and thoughts on Your Word and seek to remind me that this difficult season shall pass. Despite how bad it seems I trust that You have it in Your control. *~Deborah Farmer*

Remembering To Laugh

"A cheerful heart is good medicine…" (Proverbs 17:22a).

A friend of mine copes from severe chronic back pain, and as she walked down the hallway at church, an acquaintance asked, "How are you doing?" She prefers not to answer "fine," since she is often in pain; she wants to add a bit of truth. She answered, "I'm hanging in there."

The man quickly replied, "Like a strawberry in Jello ®?" The visual image that this brought to her was enough to stop her in her tracks, and she burst out laughing. It has been some time since she shared this with me, and I still smile when I picture that strawberry.

Science has proven that laughter and humor increases our ability to fight pain, but God knew this way before the scientist Norman Cousins discovered it. There are days when it can be difficult to see the humor in our lives. Laughter may not come as spontaneously or as often as it once did, and this is when it becomes vital, for both our health and our emotions, to search it out. Take a moment to look for the humor in your activities, and if you can't find it, create it.

- Give yourself a gold star for everything you do today.
- Dunk your cookies.
- Dot all your i's with smiley faces.
- Sing into your hairbrush.
- Have a staring contest with your cat.
- Eat ice cream for breakfast.
- Blow the wrapper off a straw.
- Refuse to eat crusts.
- Make a face the next time somebody tells you "no."
- Ask "Why?" a lot.
- Have someone read you a story.
- Wear your favorite shirt with your favorite pants even if they don't match.

Lord, don't allow me to take life too seriously. Even You know, "A cheerful heart is good medicine," (Proverbs 17:22). ~Lisa Copen

God Never Withers

"All men are like grass, and all glory is like the flowers of the field; the grass withers and the flowers fall, but the Word of the Lord stands forever," (1 Peter 1:24-25).

I enjoy taking my dog on a walk through our neighborhood park, listening to the birds and eyeing the gorgeous flowers. One particular beautiful spring day, I noticed a special bunch of blue flowers in the corner of a yard. They were bluebonnets, the state flower of Texas. Glistening in the bright Texas sun, they smelled of fresh air and sweet perfume. How God's creation proclaims His glory!

As I rode past them in my electric wheelchair, the phrase "Bloom where you are planted" came to my mind. Jeremiah 24:16 says, "I will plant them and not uproot them." We are "planted" by God in order to declare the Glory of the Loving, Sovereign Lord, through our lives, in whatever "corner" of the world He chooses to put us. How pretty these bluebonnets were, growing in this corner of the yard, standing out from the freshly cut green grass.

Just days later, I went past that same yard, and those beautiful flowers had withered and died. The words of Peter are so true. "The grass withers and the flowers fall, but the Word of the Lord stands forever," (1 Peter 1:24-25). Elisabeth Elliot, author and teacher, says, "God is God. Because He is God, He is worthy of my trust and obedience. I will find rest nowhere but in His holy will, a will that is unspeakably beyond my largest notions of what He is up to."[21]

What a comfort is the verse in 1 Peter. God's Word is everlasting, standing forever. In this world we see pain, sorrow, and death, but the eternal Word of God will never die.

Lord, help me to study my Bible daily. You use it to comfort, console, convict, and encourage me. *~Holly Baker*

I Don't Feel Very Pretty

"Those who look to Him are radiant," (Psalm 34:5a).

When a chronic illness enters our lives, it is easy for our self-image to become affected. We have less energy. We feel less attractive. Our fewer visible achievements make us feel less valuable. Our bodies feel like they are turning against us, and we feel betrayed. Dreams are dwindling.

Pain also isolates us. When we feel unwell, we are less likely to be involved with other people. We choose to put on the clothes that are most comfortable, rather than current styles. We go days without makeup. What's the use in getting fixed up just to be alone in the house all day?

It is in times like this that my relationship with Christ also suffers. It is as though I choose to take the easy way out of everything. . . and that includes my time with Him. Sometimes I feel like it's all His fault. He's the one that took so much away from me! I would be successful if it weren't for the illness. I would be stylish if it weren't for the pain. I would be attractive if it weren't for the side effects of the medication. I could concentrate on Him more fully.

When I get to this state, however, I must remind myself that I am not seeing myself as God sees me. Regardless of my body's abilities or its appearance, I am still His child, and that makes me beautiful. Psalm 34:5a says, "Those who look to Him are radiant." "Radiance" means shining, brilliant, beaming, and sparkling. That's a far cry from unwashed hair and baggy sweats. When we look to Him, His radiance is reflected on our face. I've got to run. . . my curling iron is hot!

Lord, how You see me is all that really matters. Of course, when I imagine what You must truly see in me, I feel a bit more motivated to let others see this sparkling me that is just waiting to get out. I want to represent You well, Lord. Let my spirit glow.

~Lisa Copen

He's Got It Under Control

"God is our refuge and strength, an ever-present help in trouble. Therefore we will not fear, though the earth give way and the mountains fall into the heart of the sea, though its waters roar and foam and the mountains quake with their surging," (Psalm 46:1, 2).

My husband and I are pursuing adoption, and our constant fear has been, "What if a birth mom changes her mind and we have to give the baby back?" Everyone is quick to share the nightmare stories they have heard. After we left our second adoption meeting, however, we both felt a profound peace about the entire situation. *Nothing* could happen to us that was not Father-filtered.

If a mom changed her mind, it would only mean that God had a better plan. Of course, it would hurt more than I could imagine; but because of our faith, we would be able to move ahead, rather than become depressed and hopeless.

So it is with our illness. We have all experienced these quakes and rumbles explained in Psalm 46:2 in our own lives. Some of us remember the day the doctor said, "You have an illness called — ." Others would simply like to hear any diagnosis because they are exhausted with not being able to figure out what is happening to their body. Our lives crumble at times. Families break apart. Friendships deteriorate. Our health continues to falter. So what *is it* that keeps us alive and even joyful? Knowing that we have nothing to fear gives us the ability to keep moving forward with hope and confidence. We are able to enjoy even the small moments in life simply because we recognize them as a gift.

God, I understand that things may not work out exactly as I would prefer. In fact, I know they likely will not. However, I do have Your promise that You will take care of me every step of the way and that Your plan is always perfect. ~*Lisa Copen*

Pass It On

"Praise be to God, the Father of our Lord Jesus Christ, the Father of compassion and the God of all Comfort, who comforts us in all of our troubles, so that we can comfort those in any trouble with the comfort we ourselves have received from God," (2 Corinthians 1:3,4).

As a youngster, I went Bible camp during summer months. I remember singing songs around the campfire, and I was the loudest singer when my favorite song came up, *"Pass It On."* "It only takes a spark to get a fire going, and soon all those around can warm up in its glowing...."[22] As a young adult, I taught this song to my church youth choir; as a mom, I passed it on to my kids.

We can pass on God's love to others who are in need. With my body pierced with pain, it is harder to be cheerful in song. Hurt and depression can control my emotions, making it difficult to imagine myself passing on comfort to others.

However, we are reminded that God loves us so much that He has compassion on us. He can be our source of comfort when times are hard. We can praise God for carrying us through the troubled waters. He promises to empower us with endurance if we trust Him in faith. When we realize that it is our Heavenly Father who has sustained and empowered us through His compassion and love for us, we can then comfort another hurting soul by sharing this revelation with them. We can pass on God's love and, in doing so, strengthen our faith and endurance to help us cope in the midst of our own troubles. You are so loved.

Albert Schweitzer once said, "Sometimes our light goes out but is blown into flame by another human being. Each of us owes deepest thanks to those who have rekindled this light."[23]

Lord, let my life be a testimony that will empower another one who is suffering. It only takes a spark! *~Deborah Farmer*

God's Everlasting Presence

"The Lord, He is the One who goes before you. He will be with you, He will not leave you nor forsake you; do not fear nor be dismayed," (Deuteronomy 31:8).

Do you have moments when your illness-related circumstances are impossible to accept? All of the associated concerns of medicine, insurance, doctors visits and lack of understanding from others often overwhelms us more than the pain itself. Circumstances seem out of our control.

God reminds us in 2 Corinthians 4:17, "For our light and momentary troubles are achieving for us an eternal glory that far outweighs them all." We suffer daily, and our illnesses are heavy burdens, but we must remind ourselves that, compared to eternity, they are "light and momentary." Depression may come, but comfort will too, when we learn to deal with these frustrations day by day, dwelling on the Word of God and the power of the Holy Spirit. God will not leave us or forsake us even when we feel despair. I've heard the saying, "The shortest distance between a problem and a solution is the distance between your knees and the floor."

In *The Storm Within*, Mark Littleton writes, "If you are caught in an endless cycle of pain that seems unending, dark, a veritable pit, take heart in the fact that you don't have to be joyful to 'count' as a Christian. Your testimony has not been shattered. You are not a 'poor excuse' for a Christian or an example of 'unconfessed sin.' If you are enduring, if you are sticking with it despite your pain, you are achieving, as Paul saying, an overwhelming victory," (See Romans 8:37).[24]

Lord, You do hear my cry. Although I may not "feel" Your presence, You are there, guiding my steps. "But as for me, I will always have hope; I will praise You more and more," (Psalm 71:14). This means I will wait with expectancy, that I will be patient for that which will come. *~Patricia Armstrong*

Following The Crowd

"We all, like sheep, have gone astray, each of us has turned to his own way," (Isaiah 53:6a)

Bored Royal Air Force pilots stationed on the Falkland Islands devised what they thought was a wonderful game. Noting that the local penguins seemed fascinated by airplanes, the pilots flew their planes slowly along the water's edge as nearly ten thousand penguins turned their heads in unison, watching the planes go by. To give the penguins a little variety, the pilots flew out to sea, turned around, and flew over the top of the penguin colony. Once again, in unison, heads went up, up, up, until all ten thousand penguins toppled softly onto their backs.[25] How much simpler it is to go along with the crowd! Sometimes we blindly follow one another regardless of where we are led. "We all, like sheep, have gone astray…" (Isaiah 53:6a).

Living with chronic illness can make us feel alone and isolated; we are no longer able to flock with the crowd. Perhaps we have given up our walking buddies or skipped shopping for hours at a time. Our friends talk about the stresses of their careers; we feel useless, as we struggle just to take a shower or hold a conversation. Some friends drift away despite our efforts to try to keep up… and it hurts.

Christ can work through any circumstance; perhaps His breaking us away from the crowd that we once flocked with is a way in which He is pruning us. If you've ever pruned a rosebush, you know that occasionally you must cut off a few blooms, maybe even buds. Perhaps a fast-paced friend was a bloom that God pruned away in order to help you continue to grow into His image. God has something better in store!

"Christ has taken up our infirmities and has carried our sorrows," (Isaiah 53:4). Remind me I have a magnificent reason for which to praise. You are molding me into something special, not just one of the crowd.

~Lisa Copen

Honor This Body?

"Do you know that your body is a temple of the Holy Spirit who is in you, whom you have received from God?" (1 Corinthians. 6:19).

Brushing my hair, I caught a glance of my hand in the mirror. It has gradually become malformed, and, although I see the changes in it every day, it somehow looks more profound in my reflection. *This is what other people see. . .* I think. *That's why they sometimes stare.* Time is not being kind to my body. It feels worn out and weathered, and I'm only thirty-four years old. What will it be like in thirty more years? Surely when God says to honor thy body, He's not talking to *us,* right? My body has done nothing but betray me over and over again. It aches, flares, and burns. Perhaps you feel the same. *Why I am still commanded to give this body respect?*

1 Corinthians 6:19-20 says, "Do you know that your body is a temple of the Holy Spirit who is in you, whom you have received from God? You are not your own. You were bought at a price. Therefore, honor God with your body." I wonder if Paul had his reasons for *asking* instead of *telling* us. "You hoo, hey there, yes you! Do *you* know?"

Grab a piece of paper and draw an outline of your body. Inside, list the words that describe your body. I know, it is not a fun exercise, but try it. I would start out with: puffy, swollen, undependable, betrayer.... Now fold it in half and write the words of 1 Corinthians 6:19-20 on the outside in big bold letters. It doesn't matter what's inside, because God has already paid a price. Your body is a *temple of the Holy Spirit.* It is filled with God, given by God, owned by God, and paid for by God. Last week I saw a mother in a wheelchair stop and demand that her young daughter get her the cigarettes out of her purse behind the chair. I could see the pain and worry in the girl's eyes. Your body is a gift to many around you too.

Lord, help me honor my body. It is a gift not just to You, but to those who love me too. *~Lisa Copen*

More Effort Equals More Joy

"A gift opens the way for the giver and ushers him into the presence of the great," (Proverbs 18:16).

One of the things I miss from my life before illness is the ease in which I could whip up a baked dessert for a party to take to friends as a surprise. Today, I decided I was going to make a peach pie. . . somehow! At first, I was tempted to buy a pie at the grocery store, but the crust didn't look nearly as appetizing as I remembered mine being. And so I went over to the produce section and bought a big bag of peaches.

It took nearly an hour to peel enough peaches for just one pie. My fingers were sore, and I could feel the tendons straining about halfway through the bagful, but I wasn't going to give up. As I peeled, I tried to think about how much I was going to enjoy the satisfaction of knowing I made a pie, despite all of the pain. I tried hard not to think about how much simpler it once was.

When my husband walked in the door, he was stunned to smell the aroma of a fresh peach pie, and he was thrilled with my efforts. Friends also appreciate the little things that we do because they know that it took more effort on our part than it may have for a healthy person. For example, I made a quilt for one of my friend's first babies, and when she opened the package, tears came to her eyes. The quilt, made with my swollen, malformed hands, was a symbol of just how much I cared about her.

Ecclesiastes 10:10 says, "If the ax is dull and its edge unsharpened, more strength is needed but skill will bring success." If the task is harder because of circumstances, the joy one will receive when it is complete will be even greater than it would have been had the task been easy to complete.

Lord, let me give a gift of sacrifice to open the door wide so that I can share about Your goodness in my life. *~Lisa Copen*

I Am So Discouraged

"'For I know the plans I have for you,' declares the Lord, 'plans to prosper you and not harm you, plans to give you hope and a future. Then you will call upon Me, and I will listen to you,'" (Jeremiah 29:11,12).

My entire life, I have been learning how to become emotionally vulnerable; it is one of the reasons I suffer from clinical depression. Since becoming more vulnerable, however, my feelings are more raw. Friends and loved ones, who I thought would be here when I needed them, have deserted me. I truly don't understand it. If they were going through a crisis, I would be there for them. Little has changed in our world since Job uttered these words to his friends: "You too have proved to be of no help. You see something dreadful and are afraid," (Job 6:21). If illness has "gotten me," surely it can get them too!

Do you find yourself alone? We often hear friends tell us, "If you'd stop thinking about how poorly you feel, you will feel better!" or "Stop wallowing in self-pity and think about what you do have!" Perhaps, all you want is for someone to reach out to you and listen, someone to empathize.

So, where does it leave those of us who are hurting and in pain? It brings us to God the Father. God knows the deep wounds we face. God will never abandon us in our time of need. "And surely, I am with you always, to the very end of the age," (Matthew 28:20). He understands what we are going through and weeps along with us when we are hurting. Jim Elliot, a missionary who paid with the price of his life, said, "I may no longer depend on pleasant impulses to bring me before the Lord. I must rather respond to principles I know to be right, whether I feel them to be enjoyable or not."

Lord, I turn to You even though I am discouraged and don't feel like it. I know You love me like no other can love me. Only You have the authentic comfort that I seek. *~Kay DeCarlo*

Are These Chains A Gift?

"As a result, it has become clear throughout the whole palace guard and to everyone else that I am in chains for Christ," (Philippians 1:13).

I weep, I whine, I scream, I plead, but the pain remains. We each have a choice: to continue in a state of dishevelment or to surrender our pain over to God and move on. As I stood up to speak at Rest Ministries' first benefit concert, I felt the power of Christ behind me saying, "They know that you are in pain and that you love Me in spite of it." It gave me such peace to be given the opportunity for people to know that, despite my personal chains, I continued to serve God. I prayed that the people who were there who were not Christians, and not in pain, would go home and ask themselves, "If a tragedy like this can enter her life and she still chooses to serve God, who is this God that provides this comfort in such pain?"

We may not like the testimony that we have been given, but pain has given each of us a form of testifying to the world that we are walking that difficult path and God is sustaining us. "Testimony" means, "we have withstood the test." Our pain gives us a natural way to bring up our faith in conversation. As I was walking the length of the pool the other day, the woman beside me, also in physical therapy, said, "The only thing that keeps me going is prayer." By the time we reached the end of the pool, we were good friends. We shared both the experience of physical pain and a relationship with our Lord. It is hard for me to bring up my pain without mentioning my faith; they go hand in hand.

Lord, teach me to use these chains to honor You and glorify You, even when they feel heavy and burdensome. Give me the opportunity to show others that my positive attitude does not come from my own strength, but from Yours. And when I don't have that positive attitude, help me remember that You have given me a gift and I am to use it wisely and with graciousness. *~Lisa Copen*

Must I Learn Obedience?

"Although He was a Son, He learned obedience from what He suffered and, once made perfect, He became the source of eternal salvation for all who obey Him," (Hebrews 5:8,9).

Sometimes I do not understand God's plan. I want to go to the women's retreat at my church, and yet the hike from the sleeping quarters to the dining room would wear me out for the day. Church is supposed to be a place of refuge, but often I am in pain. There are days when I am overwhelmed with the feeling of "this is not fair." I may have lost another ability, or cancelled plans with friends. Perhaps I have watched a tragedy on the evening news. Regardless, I am constantly reminded that we are not yet in heaven. Life here on earth is not perfect and never will be.

I am gradually learning obedience to God. To make it through the day and stay in the right frame of mind, I must surrender each day to God. I must be willing to step forward to do His work when He calls me to it, and even more difficult, I must be willing to rest when He says, "Rest." Obedience is not a fun character trait to learn. I would much rather focus on joy or peace; even wisdom could have moments of glory, but learning obedience is like being on God's pottery block every day, and allowing Him to sculpt, chisel, and put me in the furnace. I'm tired of being a lump.

When these moments become difficult, I rely on Hebrews 5:8,9. "Although He was a Son, *He learned obedience from what He suffered* and, once made perfect, He became the source of eternal salvation for all who obey Him." Jesus Himself wasn't let off the hook! If He had to suffer in order to learn obedience from God, why should I be any different? The struggles I have, as I learn to obey God and listen for His voice, are all a part of His plan to shape me into His desire.

Thank You, Lord, for caring more for my everlasting spirit than for my fleshly comfort. ~*Lisa Copen*

I Feel So Defeated, Lord

"I was young and now I am old, yet I have never seen the righteous forsaken . . . . " (Psalm 37:25a).

Everywhere around me I see defeat. One man was just denied surgery because he was not a good candidate, making survival for him unlikely. A woman was told by the specialist that her lab tests make it appear as if she should not be alive, and he said, "I only treat the living." Car problems, financial struggles, and ending relationships abound throughout the group of chronically ill friends I hold dear. *Why, Lord? Why must they suffer so?* The world seems to be turning against us, and I want to brew in my discouragement and emotions of defeat.

David felt this same way much of the time. While David had feelings of discouragement, defeat, fear, and even disobedience, God never left his side. When David doubted that even God could help him, God remained with him, offering forgiveness. In a world that relies on success, materialistic items, and reputation, we are quick to feel discouraged when we don't measure up. When those around us are hurting and we don't see God intervening, we feel defeated and even betrayed. God has *never* forsaken you, and God *never will* forsake you. "Most of the verses written about praise in God's Word," says Joni Eareckson Tada, "were voiced by people faced with crushing heartaches, injustice, treachery, slander, and scores of other difficult situations."[26]

In time, we will be able to look at our life and see that, regardless of our circumstances, God prevailed. He never left us. We may have had moments of anger, frustration, and even disobedience, but our Father was always there beside us, waiting for us to invite Him back into our daily life.

God, You promise I will never see the righteous forsaken. I am hurting beyond comfort of any kind, but I won't let You go. You are the only thing I can count on unconditionally. ~Lisa Copen

God Always Provides A Light

"You, O Lord, keep my lamp burning; my God turns my darkness into light," (Psalm 18:28).

Seventy-year-old George went for his annual physical. All of his tests results were normal. Dr. Smith said, "George, everything looks great physically. How are you doing mentally and emotionally? Are you at peace with yourself, and do you have a good relationship with your God?"

George replied, "God and me are tight. He knows I have poor eyesight, so he's fixed it so that when I get up in the middle of the night to go to the bathroom, poof! The light goes on, and when I'm done, poof! The light goes off."

"Wow," commented Dr. Smith, "That's incredible!" A little later in the day Dr. Smith called George's wife. "Thelma," he said, "George is just fine. Physically he's great. I'm in awe of his relationship with God. Is it true that he gets up during the night and poof! The light goes on in the bathroom and then poof! The light goes off?"

Thelma exclaimed, "That old fool! He's peeing in the refrigerator again!"[27]

The Greeks had a unique race in their Olympic games; the winner was not the runner who finished first, but the runner who finished with his torch still lit. We're often more concerned with the I-wants than with the journey. There's a fall season in San Diego when I want to light candles to create a homey atmosphere once the sun goes down. At the same time, the air conditioner still comes on, flickering the candles. I have to choose—do I blow out the candles or turn off the air? I can't have it both ways. The illnesses in our lives can cause every bit of light within us to flicker and blow, attempting to put out our flame for Christ.

God, I can't have it both ways; I have to rid myself of some of life's luxuries and follow Christ in order to keep Your light burning. "Your word is a lamp to my feet and a light for my path," (Psalm 119:105). Poof! Turn my light on! ~*Lisa Copen*

My Mustard Seed

"It is like a mustard seed, which is the smallest seed you plant in the ground. Yet when planted, it grows and becomes the largest of all garden plants, with such big branches that the birds of the air can perch in its shade," (Mark 4:31-32).

I planted tiny seeds in my garden. The Lord supplied me with the soil, nutrients, water, and sunshine. With time and patience, lovely plants soon came from the ground, ready for harvest. Although I love to garden, my garden is quite tiny because my illness keeps me from doing too much.

Some days I feel like those tiny seeds. I am so weak and feeble. I feel like I don't have much to offer. The pain is so consuming that I am not physically able to do a whole lot. I wonder, "Am I just a weak seed? What can I do?"

When I give the Lord the seeds of my life to plant, He can use my fragile self. I am part of His huge garden. He sees the whole bountiful harvest when all I can see are those weak tiny seeds.

I have a purpose in God's plan. Perhaps it is to pray for you or encourage someone else in pain today. All I know is that this encourages me to fight another day and invites me to put my trust the Lord. You see, He understands my turmoil. He can bless those tiny seeds.

Are you suffering today? Do you feel discouraged? Do you feel that you cannot do what you once could do? Don't lose faith, dear child. Hold on to the mustard seed. The Lord knows what we are going through, and He will supply whatever nutrients or circumstances we need to fulfill His plan for our life. You are not alone today.

Lord, I am part of Your bigger plan. "For you have been born again, not of perishable seed, but of imperishable, through the living and enduring word of God," (1 Peter 1:23). ~Deborah Farmer

God Is Not Surprised

"For He knew how we are formed. He remembers that we are dust," (Psalm 103:14).

When one is diagnosed with an illness, everything in life becomes uncertain. We didn't expect this illness to enter into our life and redefine everything that we determined as "normal." Yet, God is not surprised.

Psalm 139:14-16: "I praise You because I am fearfully and wonderfully made. Your works are wonderful, I know that full well. My frame was not hidden from You when I was made in the secret place. When I was woven together in the depths of the earth, Your eyes saw my unformed body. All the days ordained for me were written in Your Book before one of them came to be." God describes our body as fearfully and wonderfully made and woven together. On those days when I feel as though everything is spinning out of my control, I must rely on God's words. He is not surprised. He knew that our future would hold this challenge. *He knew* and is working in our life to prepare us for wherever this journey will take us. Our body, as well as our soul, is in His hands.

Of course, sometimes I wish that God had allowed me to know when I was young that I would someday have an illness. Perhaps I would have lived better, harder, or more enthusiastically, but only He had the knowledge that pain would one day enter into my life and become a constant uninvited companion. Thankfully, God is my other companion, and He promises never to leave my side, regardless of circumstances, my attitude, my doubts, or my worries. He's there beside you too, waiting for you to reach out.

God, remind me that I am not living out Your "runner-up plan." You knew all along that this would be my life. I am still in Your "Plan A" for my life. Let me embrace it. I've got nothing to lose and everything to gain. *~Lisa Copen*

Giving Grace

"Be wise in the way you act toward outsiders; make the most of every opportunity. Let your conversation be always full of grace, seasoned with salt, so that you may know how to answer everyone," (Colossians 4:5,6).

I was having a painful day, and I decided to use my placard and park in a disabled parking space. The woman walking by glared as I was getting out of my car. I was relieved when she walked past, but then she turned and came back and accusingly said, "You don't look handicapped to me!"

After five years, every time I park in a disabled spot, I have to be prepared to defend this privilege I wish I didn't have. When someone approaches me, I want to scream and then cry. It was difficult for me to accept my condition and get the placard. I would quickly give up parking privileges to feel normal again. The media continues to feature exposēs of people who abuse parking privileges, provoking more of our society to take things into their own hands and approach people who have invisible illnesses. So I understand her perspective, but I still resent her judgment.

When people say, "You don't look handicapped," I am tempted to reply, "Well. . .you don't look stupid." Instead, I must remember that God has commanded me to use this opportunity to have a conversation full of grace. I must extend God's grace to the individual who doesn't understand. I may be the only Jesus they see.

I'm always eager to explain my illness and try to help others understand. The problem is, they are rarely interested in hearing about it. They would much rather criticize and walk away. I suppose that's why grace is what it is. If grace were easy to disburse, it wouldn't be worth very much.

Lord, let me be merciful. I may be the only reflection of Christ they ever see. I want to make You proud, Father. ~*Lisa Copen*

Breaking Those Chains

"Some sat in darkness and the deepest gloom, prisoners suffering in iron chains. . .. Then they cried to the Lord in their trouble, and He saved them from their distress. He brought them out of darkness and the deepest gloom and broke away their chains," (Psalm 107:10,13-14).

Have you ever been in the place that David, the Psalmist and later King of Israel, describes above? I have. It can be an extremely frightening place to reside. Perhaps, this psalm describes where you are today. Sometimes, we can go for a long time with what one writer has called, "the dark night of the soul."

I recall lying on the bed one day, my soul so very dark. Jesus promises us that He will never leave us, and yet I felt deserted by Him. I was not aware that, although I could not hold onto Him, He was holding onto me. I could only pray "Jesus, pray for me," and He did. I could not pray for myself, but Jesus prayed for me.

Beloved, are you going through the "dark night of the soul?" It can be a distressing place to be, but there is hope. For our Bible says that, when they cried to the Lord, that He brought them out of the darkness and He broke away the chains. In Acts 16:25,26, about midnight (the darkest hour), Paul and Silas were praying and singing hymns to God. "Suddenly there was such a violent earthquake that the foundations of the prison were shaken. At once all the prison doors flew open, and everybody's chains came loose."

"Jesus Christ is the same yesterday and today, and forever," (Hebrews 13:8). Those before us have prayed, sang praises, and called out to You, and You heard them and set them free. Some glorious day You are going to set me free from my pain. My prison doors are going to spring open. And the longer that I have had to wait, the more joyous this occasion will be! ~Virginia Ganskie

I Am So Grateful

"Man is a mere phantom as he goes to and fro. He bustles about, but only in vain. . . ." (Psalm 39:6,7).

I went to coffee with a friend I hadn't seen in some time. As usual, she spent a great deal of our time telling me how unhappy she is with her house and how she wants to move. She lives in a beautiful home in a neighborhood I will never be able to afford. I once sympathized with her predicaments, as she has not had an easy life; but over time, I continue to see her in a constant state of dissatifaction regardless of her circumstances. Luke 6:24 tells us, "Woe to you who are rich, for you have already received your comfort."

A part of me wonders if I too would have been on this path of discontent had it not been for getting an illness in my early twenties. I quickly discovered that I should not to take one moment of life for granted. Although I don't have all of the material items that would make my life simpler, I am completely satisfied, and consistently grateful for the blessings which God has provided. The career I was going to have did not materialize. I have yet to see all of the money I was going to make. Owning a home was more of a fantasy than a goal for many years. It is hard not to become resentful of others who have so much and yet don't appreciate it.

"What causes fights and quarrels among you? Don't they come from your desires that battle within you? You want something, but don't get it. You kill and covet, but you cannot have what you want. You quarrel and fight. You do not have, because you do not ask God. When you ask, you do not receive, because you ask with wrong motives, that you may spend what you get on your pleasures," (James 4:1-3).

Lord, thank You for using my illness as a way of saving me from my transgressions. You have used my illness as a filter, and whatever is unimportant flows right through my life.

~Lisa Copen

Searching For Your "Special Gifts"

"'Build up, build up, prepare the road! Remove the obstacles out of the way of My people.' For this is what The High and Lofty One says, He Who lives forever, Whose Name is Holy: 'I live in a high and holy place, but also with him who is contrite and lowly in spirit, to revive the spirit of the lowly and revive the heart of the contrite,'" (Isaiah 57:14,15).

I love to walk on the beach, especially the beaches of Cape Cod. Ever since I was a young girl, I would walk on the beach and feel one with God. I would always look for my special gift that the ocean would bring. Sometimes, it would be the formation of the sand, a butterfly landing on my shoulder, or a shell, but I always knew that God would speak to me in a special way. My husband and I recently went to the cape, and I discovered this trip's special gift, a conch shell. It is broken, showing only the inner portion. How much this shell represents me; it is a beautiful milky-orange color with edges smoothed by the salt and sand of the ocean, almost like porcelain. I knew this shell was left by the tide just for me.

Like the conch that is weathered by the ocean, God can take those of us weathered by chronic illness and build us up once more. Jesus said, "Blessed are those who are poor in spirit, for theirs is the Kingdom of heaven,'" (Matthew 5:3). When we realize how weak we are, how can we *not* turn our life over to God? He is waiting with open arms, desiring to open the portals of His Kingdom of Heaven to each of us, where we shall find peace and rest.

Like the broken shells, you too have value. The molding of the shell was formed by the many grains of sand that ate away at the edges until it went from being a sharp edged tool to a work of art.

God, You can and will use me if I allow You to. With a lowly spirit and contrite heart, I give myself to You. I feel so lost, so lead me and guide me every step of the way. ~*Kay DeCarlo*

His Understanding Has No Limits

"Great is our Lord and mighty in power; His understanding has no limit," (Psalm 147:5).

There are days I feel isolated in a world of pain, lost dreams, and questions about the future, and there is no one to talk with that truly can say, "I know exactly what you mean." It is during these times I turn to the Lord, who promises me that He will always be there to comfort me and that He understands the pain, the isolation, and the fears I feel. "Great is our Lord and mighty in power; His understanding has no limit," (Psalm 147:5). I sometimes catch myself looking at people and thinking "They just don't understand." This is a sign that I need to quickly refocus and put my thoughts on a loving God who *does* understand and will always be available to listen to me and give guidance.

Margaret Mitchell wrote in *Gone with the Wind*, "Life is under no obligation to give us what we expect."[28] Most of us have lived the proof of this! We can, however, know that God is faithful and reflect on the wonderful ways that He has come through for us in the past. "I remember the days of long ago; I meditate on all Your works and consider what Your hands have done," (Psalm 143:5). If you have yet to experience a history of God's faithfulness, anticipate it, count on it, and lean on it, because soon you will have a memory book of God being your protector and the driver of your life.

We all will come to the "pit of despair" in our lives, and then we will look up. Who will be there to pull us up, every time, regardless of how deep, dark, or dreary our pit is? Only Jesus. We are warned to never count on mankind to save us: "Do not put your trust in princes, in mortal men, who cannot save," (Psalm 146:3), but rather on God.

Lord, help me to surrender over to You my desire to have someone understand. Only You will be able to slip inside this body and my heart and give me the peace and understanding I seek. ~Lisa Copen

Need Dunking?

"I applied my heart to what I observed and learned a lesson from what I saw," (Proverbs 24:32).

My four-year-old cousin was dipping his cookie in his milk. "They're good, huh?" asked his mom.

"Yes," he replied. "But these cookies are so hard, I have to keep baptizing them and baptizing them."

Ever feel like you are being dunked one too many times? Living with a chronic illness can harden our shell on the outside. Physical pain makes me want to curl up; the body gradually begins to move inward, following the intuition of safety being nearer to my soul. Life has become one long instruction of, "Please keep your arms inside the moving vehicle at all times." It is not hard to understand how our spiritual life can follow suit and move inward, closer to our own pity party and away from the Lord.

It is tough being a Christian, and let us admit, it is even tougher being a Christian in pain. Nonbelievers question what's so great about being a Christian if we aren't exempt from illness. Believers ask, "Are you sure you have enough faith? Maybe you aren't praying right." It is natural to separate ourselves from gatherings that upset us. Not only are vacations more difficult, just getting to church becomes an agonizing morning. Hence, we start getting dunked! God's desire is to soften us up. He wants us to be Christ-like, not crisp-like! Last week my heart was not into attending a gathering of friends. My husband and I were one of the first to try to have children; now they have many, while we still wait to adopt. I tried to hold it together. We talked, they prayed, tears flowed. Had I remained hardened and not gone, I wouldn't have experienced their compassion.

Lord, I know I need to be dunked now and then to soften up my heart. Help me seek to recognize Your purposes. *~Lisa Copen*

Hurt When Others Hurt

"Rejoice with those who rejoice; mourn with those who mourn," (Romans 12:15).

Sometimes it's so easy to get caught up in all of my own hurts that I forget to hurt with others. Having an illness has brought me a greater sense of compassion, and yet I still struggle with not inwardly comparing others' struggles to my own. It is hard to listen when one is drained. I heard of one woman who called her circle of friends "her caseload." It is much easier to believe, "I have enough worries of my own. I don't need to hear the worries of others." It is also tempting to think, "If she had my troubles, then she'd have something to be upset about!" Like Job says, "He feels but the pain of his own body and mourns only for himself." (Job 14:22).

Romans 12:15 says, "Rejoice with those who rejoice; mourn with those who mourn." We are to do our best to *feel* what the other person is feeling. When one hurts, we are supposed to hurt with her, not compare our own problems and tell her how good she has it. Just as we are called to mourn with others, we are called to rejoice with them. Many days we must make the choice to rejoice because we don't feel joyful. When your sister tells you about her new job, you should rejoice with her, not complain about how your career was ruined by your illness. When a friend shares that she's pregnant, God wants you to rejoice, not have a bitter heart of jealousy.

Having this kind of attitude doesn't just happen. It is only by walking with Jesus each day that we are able to become more like Him. Jesus walked alongside those who were hurting. He recruited people that society had tossed aside, to help Him save lives for eternity.

Father, You knew how to hurt with someone, not just for someone. Teach me to put my problems aside for today and comfort a hurting friend with grace and intimacy. *~Lisa Copen*

Do Christians Panic?

"He shall say: 'Hear, O Israel, today you are going into battle against your enemies. Do not be fainthearted or afraid; do not be terrified or give way to panic before them,'" (Deuteronomy 20:3).

Living with bipolar and panic disorder is difficult. At times when I am anxious, I want to run and hide, my heart pounds, palms get clammy, and my chest races as my mind is filled with anxiety, panic, and sometimes despair. Reaching out, it seems no one understands this private pain we face. I feel trapped in a dark cave, with no way out.

What do I do? Pray. He is sometimes just a small flicker of hope, but just what I need. I truly do not have any control over what I face nor what will happen to me. God tells us not to be fainthearted nor afraid, for today we are going into battle against our enemies, and we are not to give way to panic before them. How do we cope? With God by our side.

We must turn to the Lord God in prayer even when we don't feel His presence. The battle has been already been won by Him. To get over this fear, we must daily acknowledge that nothing is going to happen to us that we and the Lord God Almighty cannot handle together. Listen to His command: "Have I not commanded you? Be strong and courageous. Do not be terrified, for the Lord your God will be with you wherever you go," (Joshua 1:9).

You are not alone, Beloved. God walks with you always. He understands our deepest fears and doesn't think any less of us for feeling them. He felt pain, panic, and the despair of dying—but He felt it so that we can hope even when we feel it. We have a Savior to identify with when panic and anxiety arise.

In doing so, "Though you search for your enemies, you will not find them. Those who wage war against you will be as nothing at all," (Isaiah 41:12).

~Kay DeCarlo

Returning Yourself To God

"If you return to the Lord, then your brothers and children will be shown compassion by their captors and will come back to this land, for the Lord your God is gracious and compassionate. He will not turn His face from you if you return to Him," (2 Chronicles 30:9).

Living with heart disease is difficult. Being forty years old and struggling with normal tasks, like laundry, is emotionally difficult. Some days, I can walk the half-mile around my neighborhood without problems; other days, a trip to the basement to bring up laundry leaves me huffing and puffing. Then I realize that I do have a serious illness and my heart is enlarged. I need to take a break. It's discouraging.

Do we really find rest? Do you find rest for your body and your soul, or do you lash out in anger toward God? Do you know that God is loving and compassionate, or do you blame Him for your situation? Yes, God is the God of all mankind, and nothing is impossible for Him, (Jeremiah 32:27). He cannot and will not break His own law, which is free will. He wants you to go to Him to ask for help. He won't barge in.

Beloved, God is as near as your shadow. All you need to do is be open, honest, and ask for His help. You may feel an inner peace, your heart warming up, or internal spiritual weakness being strengthened. You may find affliction, but God goes with you always. He promises, "A bruised reed He will not break, and a smoldering wick He will not snuff out. In faithfulness, He will bring forth justice," (Isaiah 42:3).

If you're unsure how to call out to God, go to Him as a child, simple in prayer and in faith.

"You hear, O Lord, the desire of the afflicted; You encourage them, and listen to their cry, defending the fatherless and the oppressed, in order that man, who is of the earth, may terrify no more," (Psalm 10:17-18). God, hear my cry. Console me with Your love.

~Kay DeCarlo

Simple Words Mean So Much

"Pleasant words are a honeycomb, sweet to the soul and healing to the bones," (Proverbs 16:24).

Every now and then someone says just the right thing. It may be something funny that makes me burst out laughing. It may be words of comfort or simple reassurance during a difficult time. Regardless, I am amazed at the difference that those perfect words can make in my day.

When my husband told me tonight, "You look really good in that outfit," something inside me squealed. When my parents tell me, "We are so proud of what you're doing," a part of me glows. When a friend notices that I have had my hair cut, I feel special. It takes just ordinary, simple, honest words to make one feel extraordinary.

The Proverb says, "Pleasant words are sweet to the soul and healing to the bones." Although my bones aren't healed by friendly words, they do feel soothed. My spirit feels soothed. The pain doesn't seem quite so unbearable. For a moment, I can forget the pain and have a sense of carefreeness that I rarely have experienced since I became ill.

Henry Drummond, an ordained minister in the late 1800's, said, "Instead of allowing yourself to be unhappy, just let your love grow as God wants it to grow. Seek goodness in others. Love more persons more—love them more impersonally, more unselfishly, without thought of return. The return, never fear, will take care of itself."[29]

God, let me remember how soothing kind words feel and help me make an effort to disburse them more often. Although I can't do a lot physically, little things make the most difference when done with Your love. I know how isolating it can be to have a chronic illness, so let me use this knowledge to make a difference in the lives of others.

~Lisa Copen

God Works It Out In The End

"At that time Jesus, full of joy through the Holy Spirit, said, 'I praise You, Father, Lord of heaven and earth, because You have hidden these things from the wise and learned, and revealed them to little children. Yes, Father, for this was Your good pleasure,'" (Luke 10:21).

Father and son stood at the cash register of the gas station, paying their bill. A cup on the counter mesmerized the little boy. We have all seen them—the cups usually have a sign taped on them that say something like, "Give a Penny. Take a Penny." As they walked toward the door, the boy took his father's hand and gave it a tug. "I don't understand," he told his dad. Confused, the father asked him what he meant. "If you give a penny and take a penny, then no one actually gets a penny. Right?" Smiling, the dad explained why it was there and how it worked. Not satisfied, the boy shook his head. "It still seems silly to me!"

Psalm 55:22 says, "Cast your cares on the Lord and He will sustain you; He will never let the righteous fall." God says we are to cast our cares on Him and to give them away to Him. We are good at setting our cares down before Him, but just before we leave His presence, we grab for our bag of worries and plop them over our backs. We unload in prayer only to reload again. It is no surprise that we have problems feeling free from our burdens.

According to an old Swedish proverb, worry gives a small problem a big shadow. We feel bound in pain, chronic illness, and sin. As the child above said, in his little wisdom, it seems silly. Like the little cup on the counter, God is prepared to hold our worries if we will just lay them down and leave them there. If we do not, the process comes to nothing.

Lord, You will not forcibly take from my hands what I am not willing to lay down. You will not intrude. You are my Sustainer, waiting to help me get rid of the shadows. *~Rebecca Koszalinski*

Heaven Is A Party I Won't Miss!

"Therefore my heart is glad and my tongue rejoices; my body also will rest secure," (Psalm 16:9).

I really wanted to go to the party. Months ago, I was told to put the date on my calendar. I was excited to get the invitation in the mail last week. I even bought a new outfit. Yet, now that the party has finally arrived, here I lay in bed.

There are many days where I feel the pain and go out anyway, but today was not to be one of them. Today was one of those days when my body had a mind of its own and no amount of positive thinking was going to change its ability to function. I get so frustrated when I miss out on these precious moments of life.

Would it really have messed up Your plans so badly, Lord, if I'd been able to enjoy myself for a few hours? It is times like this I can sit and feel sorry for myself, or I can think about what God has promised. Revelation 21:4 says, "He will wipe every tear from their eyes. There will be no more death or mourning or crying or pain, for the old order of things has passed away."

My time will come. Your time will come. We are going to sit around at cafes with golden tables and talk about old times here on earth. We'll pass around photos of the bodies we left behind and laugh about how they never seemed to behave when we depended on them. I'll truly know I am in heaven when I can play volleyball in high heels. (And I will finally get the ball over the net!)

"When you are on your beds, search your hearts and be silent," (Psalm 4:4).

Okay, Lord, for now I am to be in this bed and not at the party. But I hope You have angels hanging up streamers and putting up my volleyball net, because heaven is going to be one party I am not going to miss!

~Lisa Copen

Cancer Isn't Sexy

"'For your Maker is your husband; the Lord Almighty is His name. The Holy One of Israel is your Redeemer; He is called the God of all the earth. The Lord will call you back as if you were a wife deserted and distressed in spirit; a wife who married young, only to be rejected,' says your God," (Isaiah 54:5,6).

I am in my fifth month of cancer treatment, and my husband and I find our selves discussing physical intimacy more frequently. I do not doubt my husband's love for me, but I do feel we are merely coexisting right now. Let's face it: I am bald! My once shapely body has changed with the weight loss. It's hard to feel attractive, and it is so hot to wear a hat, let alone a wig, around the house. In his sweet honesty, he has admitted that it has been very difficult for him. In return, I'm missing the touch, the romance, and my self-confidence is reeling. I find myself fishing for compliments.

One morning, in his own defense of not being as attentive or affectionate, he made the shocking statement, "A lot of men just leave." This statement pierced my heart. What would I do without him? Michael is the best, a loving and generous father to our kids. He provides for us incredibly. He is almost perfect, a man who loves God and studies His Word. I am ashamed to ask for more. While searching the Scriptures for comfort, I came across Isaiah 54:5,6. *Thank You, my God.* Again He meets me where my greatest need exists; a need that seems so deep and that no one else sees, and He swoops me up in His arms. If you are married and missing your pre-illness sexual relationship, you both need to find someone with whom to talk frankly. I don't want my husband to have his mind tempted to go where it shouldn't. He is a man. He has needs. We both do. It's all a part of the journey.

Lord, please be with my spouse today. Fill him with your love, peace, and assurance of my love and appreciation. Keep my loved one from temptation. Show me what I can do for my spouse to show my appreciation. *~Norma Rose Eckblad*

I Know Too Much

"For with much wisdom comes much sorrow; the more knowledge, the more grief," (Ecclesiastes 1:18).

When Karen was told that she had lupus, she was devastated. She had been living with fears for over three months and had finally decided she could no longer avoid the tests. Her doctor apologetically gave her the bad news and told her to hang in there.

Although coming to the realization that you have an illness is never easy, it is especially difficult for Karen because she has been a nurse for over fifteen years. She has seen the effects of lupus. She has witnessed the pain. She has watched as patients lost their careers, spouses, and even their joyful spirit, because of the progression of the disease. At times such as this, she wishes she did not have medical knowledge. She would like to be ignorantly uninformed.

When we are diagnosed with an illness, it can be tempting to read every book we can find on the condition that we have. We want to know every fear that we can expect so that we can be prepared for any symptom that appears. Although it is wise to be your own medical advocate, it can also be emotionally draining to focus on descriptions such as "debilitating illness," "crippling disease," "incurable," and "terminal." These descriptions may even be out of date! And they often cause us to worry incessantly and unnecessarily.

Be informed. Do your own research. Understand your illness, but then turn it over to God and ask Him to give you wisdom, guidance, and discernment in interpreting your findings. "For with much wisdom comes much sorrow; the more knowledge, the more grief," (Ecclesiastes 1:18).

Lord, let me be discerning and responsible in the gathering and interpretation of information. Give me wisdom in order to save me from unnecessary grief. ~*Lisa Copen*

Am I In Denial?

"I will take refuge in the shadow of Your wings until the disaster has passed," (Psalm 57:1).

I was standing in front of a Rest Ministries exhibit table at a disability conference when a young woman approached me and began to share her story. It was her first time at a disability conference, and although she had lost the lower half of her leg as a child, she had never considered herself disabled. "I've waterskiied, rock climbed—I've done it all," she exclaimed. "On the way home from the hospital after my amputation my mom said, 'I don't ever want to hear you mention your leg again. Just learn to cope,' and I've been determined to do just that!"

"That's wonderful," I encouraged her. "You sound like an amazing woman."

"Yes, and I feel God calling me to be here, but I want to be here as a staff person, not as an attendee with a disability! Do you think I'm in denial? People always tell me I'm in denial."

"Well, look at the this table," I said, swooping my arm across the books I had written, the programs I had set up, and the map of two hundred HopeKeepers groups. "*This* is my form of denial. I keep busy to stay distracted from the pain."

The dictionary defines "denial" as, "a psychological defense mechanism in which confrontation with a personal problem or with reality is avoided by denying the existence of the problem or reality."[30] Denial can be an effective temporary coping mechanism, but one must turn denial into something constructive. Denial is also defined as "refusal to admit the truth or reality." Is your denial the Lord's denial or merely man's restrictions on what they consider your limitations?

Every day I deny some of the limits others have set for me, Lord. I refuse to accept dooming statistics. Only You hold my reality in Your hands. Let my denial be constructive, not destructive. Let me face reality with the hope You provide. ~*Lisa Copen*

Jesus Hears Your Deepest Cries

"Out of the depths I cry to You, O Lord. O Lord, hear my voice. Let Your ears be attentive to my cry for mercy," (Psalm 130:1,2).

Billy Graham's wife, Ruth, tells the story of the family cat that decided to have her kittens on the bed in the guest room. Not wanting them on the bed, Mrs. Graham made up a cozy bed of blankets in a box and placed it, with the kittens in it, in the kitchen.

The mother cat then proceeded to take the kittens, one by one, back to the bed in the guest room. However, she neglected to take the runt of the litter. He remained alone in the kitchen. Had she forgotten about him? Had she rejected the wee thing? Or was she just busy feeding the others?

Then the little kitten, lonesome and probably afraid, made a noise. It wasn't quite a meow; It was more of a squeak that was barely audible. Within seconds, the mother cat glided swiftly into the room, jumped in the box, grasped the kitten by the scruff of its neck, and delivered it safely to the bed in the guest room. Despite the fact that she had been two rooms, three doors, and two hallways away, the mother had heard that pitiful little squeak and come to her baby's rescue.[31]

Jesus is like that. At three o'clock in the morning, when the pain is tremendous and I just don't have the energy or the words to pray, I can just whisper the name of Jesus, and He is there. I know that when someone calls my name, I immediately turn and focus my attention on him. Jesus is no different. My friend, I encourage you, when you're tired and overwrought and words fail you, just whisper, "Jesus… Jesus," and Jesus will be there.

When I speak Your name, Jesus, no matter how weakly or how softly, You hear and immediately respond. You want to share everything with me, in good times or difficult. ~Mary Lou Cornish

God Equips The Called

"Listen, my son, to your father's instructions, and do not forsake your mother's teachings," (Proverbs 1:8).

Children are a blessing, and when I became a mother, I was excited about educating my children by the instruction of God's Word. Home schooling was my calling of ministry. Later, however, illness became a major focus, causing me to prioritize my time more effectively to carry out my responsibilities. Sometimes, despite my best efforts, disabilities interfere with my family duties. My previous, very active lifestyle is now different due to illness.

When home schooling became a challenge due to physical pain, I had to stop being a teacher and be a pupil; I placed my faith in the Lord. Many factors in the life of an educator with a chronic illness can leave one feeling weak, drained, and unable to focus. When our days seem long and shadowed, we must remember that the ultimate teacher is waiting to carry us through our trials. The Lord, who never forsakes His children, has never given people a task without equipping them with the right tools to do that task.

We may have to reprioritize our life, delegate responsibilities and simplify our home, but the Lord will provide a means for us to complete our ministry even in the midst of suffering. Through prayer and faith in God's Word, we can rest assured that our callings are not in vain regardless of our weaknesses. We can hold fast to the promise that God's Word is true by teaching the instruction of God's Word and letting our children see how we rely on Christ's strength in our home; we are giving our children the best tools to endure life's bumps and grow in the Lord.

Lord, help me feel the presence of the Holy Spirit; let me draw strength from You, the Heavenly Teacher, who loves me. Renew my passions for the ministry in which You have called me to serve.

~Deborah Farmer

What About Him?

"When Peter saw him, he asked, 'Lord, what about him?' Jesus answered, 'If I want him to remain alive until I return, what is that to you? You must follow Me,'" (John 21:21-23).

Well-known Christian author C.S. Lewis wrote *The Problem of Pain*, a book that many have turned to through the decades for answers about their suffering. What many do not know, however, is that years later, Lewis' wife passed away after a long battle with cancer. His book following her death, *A Grief Observed*, was his cry to the Lord, "Why? Why her?"

After encouraging the multitudes with his words of God's love even in the pits of suffering, I can imagine Lewis asking Jesus, "What about the others who aren't suffering? Why take my wife after all the unselfish ways we have served you?"

There are no simple answers. Christians and nonbelievers alike are both susceptible to the evil influences of the world, including chronic illnesses. As a believer, we often want to collect tangible perks for being a Christian. Sure, heaven will be a great celebration, but what about now? What about the electric bill and the ulcer?

As Christians we are given mercy, strength, peace, joy, and even patience, regardless of our circumstances. God uses the sin in the world in many ways that will bring glory to Him. We can reach out to nonbelievers and live a life that shows others that we couldn't make it without Jesus. We're also prevented from being judges of who deserves what. God knows what He will allow into who's life. We don't get to decide how to distribute the fairness around. Imagine the mess if we did! That healthy person that parked in the handicapped parking spot would be zapped with a 24-hour limp! Everything that touches our life is Father-filtered.

Lord, remind me that life isn't fair. I deserved nothing… but You gave me eternity. *~Lisa Copen*

God's Methods And Motives

"Seek the Lord while He may be found; call on Him while He is near. Let the wicked forsake his way and the evil man his thoughts. Let him turn to the Lord, and He will have mercy on him, and to our God, for He will freely pardon. 'For My thoughts are not your thoughts, neither are your ways My ways,' declares the Lord. 'As the heavens are higher than the earth, so are My ways higher than your ways and My thoughts than your thoughts,'" (Isaiah 55:6-9).

There was a man in my church who had dedicated his life to serving God, yet he was taken in a car accident. It left us all bewildered and shocked, asking, *Why?* I know I was personally stunned, for I had seen him that morning on my way to work, yet I received a call mid-afternoon to say he had died in an accident that morning.

How many times have you wondered why a particular event occurred? So often I've thought, "Why did God do it that way?" Or, "If I were God, I wouldn't have used that method!" Isaiah 55:6-9 tells us that God sees and acts from an entirely different perspective.

Jesus tells us in John 12:24, speaking of Himself, "Unless a kernel of wheat falls to the ground and dies, it remains only a single seed. But if it dies, it produces many seeds." This can also be said of followers of Jesus. Consider that, for the first few lives yielded to God, many more around this nation, and indeed around the world, have heard the Good News and placed their hope and trust in the Lord. Many have renewed their commitment to God and again focused on Him. We look at our chronic illness or pain and again ask, *Why? Haven't You got a better way, Lord? Why me?* The answer?

"'For My thoughts are not your thoughts, neither are your ways My ways,' declares the Lord. 'As the heavens are higher than the earth, so are My ways higher than your ways and My thoughts than your thoughts.'"

~Ron Cameron

A Friend Indeed

"A friend loves at all times, and a brother is born for adversity," (Proverbs 17:17).

I recently read about Vice Admiral James B. Stockdale being tortured in a Vietnamese prisoner of war camp.[32] He heard the sound of a towel snapping in the distance. It was a coded message. He and his fellow prisoners had devised ways of communicating with each other using sounds. Through his pain, Stockdale recognized a sequence of snaps spelling out GBUJS. "God bless you, Jim Stockdale." That secret message from a fellow sufferer lifted his spirits and helped him survive. "Let us not give up meeting together, as some are in the habit of doing, but let us encourage one another—and all the more as you see the day approaching," (Hebrews 10:25). "You and I may be mutually encouraged by each other's faith," (Romans 1:2).

We, who are constantly in pain and dealing with the frustrations of chronic illness, are so grateful when we have friends like folks at Rest Ministries who lift our spirits and give us encouragement. Even as we suffer, we can also be a blessing and comfort to others who are having difficult times. A friend loves at all times, especially in adversity. As we deal with our trials, let us also look for ways we can comfort others through prayer, a kind word, phone call, card, or just a word of thanks to a caretaker. Aristotle, the Greek philosopher, once said, "The best friend is the man who, in wishing me well, wishes it for my sake." True friends are selfless, but only God is truly selfless all of the time.

God is perfect love and perfect wisdom. We do not pray in order to change His Will, but to bring our wills into harmony with His.

Heavenly Father, I ask You to give me peace and to show me ways to comfort others who are also suffering. Use my circumstances to further Your perfect will. *~Patricia Armstrong*

How Much Worse Will It Get?

"No tempatation has seized you except what is common to man. And God is faithful and will not let you be tempted beyond what you can bear. But when you are tempted, He will also provide a way out so that you can stand up under it," (1 Corinthians 10:13).

Today was a really bad day. When someone asked me how I was feeling, I didn't give my standard "fine, thanks" response. Instead, I smiled and said, "Well. . . like a semi-truck just ran over me." One may believe that this sounds overdramatic, but for anyone who has lived with chronic pain, it probably sounds like an accurate description.

How much worse is God going to allow this illness to get? I wonder. *Was I not prayerful yesterday? Do I not thank Him enough for what I do have?* I am trying so hard to learn the lesson that God is teaching, but the pain continues to worsen each day. I feel too distracted by the pain to learn anything.

1 Corinthians 10:13 should comfort me, but when it took fifteen minutes to get from my bed to the shower this morning, I felt like maybe God's signals had gotten crossed; He obviously didn't get my message yesterday about reaching my limit. Mother Teresa once said, "I know that God won't give me more than I can handle. I just wish that He didn't trust me so much."

Lord, if You're listening, I just don't know how much more I can take. Just existing is becoming more painful than I ever imagined. Lord, I want my life back. I'm not demanding a cure or a healing. I'd just like to be able to function. I want to be a wife, a mom, and a friend. I want to be the "me" that is under the skin! I know that He will hear my prayer. I hope that I will get the answer I want and some of the pain will go away. If not, I have no choice but to assume that He will provide me with the strength that I need to get through one more day.

Lord, You are always faithful. *~Lisa Copen*

Our Enemies Can't Grab Us!

"The Lord will be your confidence. He will keep your foot from getting caught," (Proverbs 3:26).

Did you know there are twenty-six bones in the foot? God's precision is amazing when we think about how specialized He made us. Despite His design, the swollen, tender balls of my feet stubbornly refuse to walk to all of the places my mind and heart want to explore.

When I opened up my Bible, I laughed as I read, "The Lord will be your confidence. He will keep your foot from getting caught," (Proverbs 3:26). I remember when I wore heels and occasionally, as I walked on a sidewalk or on plank flooring, my heel would get stuck; it felt like something reached up and grabbed ahold of my whole leg. My first response was surprise or even fear, but then I would lean back into the shoe and twist my foot around until it came loose. Once in a while I'd have to casually step out of my shoe and try to gracefully pry it out of the crack, avoiding the smiles of onlookers. God's Word tells us that He will never allow our enemies or our fears to jump up and grab us. He will give us the protection we need to keep us safe from life's harms.

Where are you getting stuck? Some of us get stuck in the cycle of grief, never learning to get over the anger or the hurt. Some of us get stuck in the nobody-understands-me blues. We get stuck in the they-don't-appreciate-what-they-have-complaints. Some of us even decide that we are going to take care of ourselves, at the expense of everyone else—we send our spouses out the door on vacations without us and our children into day care—and we lose them, and they replace us… and we wonder why.

God, there are all kinds of ways I can get stuck; the enemy comes to me in many forms. It takes Your power to go up against all the stickiness. Help me choose joy, even when I don't feel like it, so that I won't ever get stuck in my circumstances. ~*Lisa Copen*

Freed from My Cage

"Then you will know the truth, and the truth will set you free," (John 8:32).

When I was a child, I loved to visit the zoo. One of my clearest memories was of a bald eagle. Eagles seem so free; the whole sky is theirs to claim. The eagle at the zoo, however, wasn't free. Locked in a cage, this magnificent creature couldn't soar to limitless heights. It just perched on a tree branch. A sign informed visitors that this eagle was unable to fly because it was blind.

There was a time when I felt like that caged eagle. I would look at myself in my wheelchair, and I felt like it was my cage. While others walked freely, I sat in my cage. I wanted so badly to soar and to ride the wind. I wanted freedom. I wondered why no one would let me out of the cage. I knew my destiny was to fly free.

Since then, I have come to realize that I resemble that eagle in the zoo more than I believed. Not only was I in a cage, I was also blind… blind to the truth that God would unlock the cage door if I just called out to Him. Once I grasped the wonderful Truth, the cage door opened, providing my life of freedom. I flew among the clouds. I rode the wind.

Some may think I'm still locked in a cage because I remain in a wheelchair. But look a little deeper. Look into my heart, and you won't see my cage. Look at my hope and joy, and you will know I'm free. With every prayer I pray, I soar. With every word I write, I'm free. With every moment placed in God's hands, I ride the wind.

Lord, am I soaring? I want to soar, regardless of my circumstances, and be able to thank You for my freedom. I don't want to be locked in a cage, unable to even stretch my wings. Show me the Truth so You can set me free. Only my uncaged soul can soar to limitless heights.

~Jason R. Mitchener

God Will Restore Your Soul

"He makes me lie down in green pastures, He leads me beside quiet waters, He restores my soul," (Psalm 23:2).

For many months prior to my dad's death, he lay in his hospital bed, unable to go outside. He would recite the words of the refreshing and restoring twenty-third Psalm. By the sound of his voice, the look in his eyes, and the serenity that shone upon his face, I knew that my earthly father was experiencing the restoration of his soul and the peace that only the Lord could give. Every time he repeated this Psalm, dad was "lying down in green pastures," right there in the living room, where his hospital bed had been placed.

I often seek refuge and solace outside, sitting on the swing nestled amongst trees in my backyard. With the recent landscaping of our backyard, the new grass that is surfacing is like velvet. This is my "green pasture," where the Lord God comes to me and restores my soul. Many of us have a special place outdoors where we can find the closeness and comfort with the Lord that restores the soul. In this special place, we are one with Him as the spirit of the living God falls fresh and new upon us, cleansing and restoring our body, mind, and spirit. If you are unable to go outdoors, He restores a soul through visual images that He plants in the mind and spirit of those who read, hear, or remember His Word.

Psalm 23:1 in *The Message* says, "God, My Shepherd! I don't need a thing." Such are the green pastures that I pray you may envision and experience each day as you allow God to restore you, in spite of, and because of, the chronic illnesses you endure.

Lord, I want to experience Your restoring love and power today as You, my Shepherd, make me lie down in green pastures and lead me beside quiet waters. With You beside me, I don't need a thing.

~Nancy Wilcox

From Hurt – To Heal!

"Is there no balm in Gilead? Is there no physician there? Why then is there no healing for the wound of My people?" (Jeremiah 8:22).

I cried, "Lord, use me!"
He answered, "Wait."
Then came the hurt.
Loneliness. I walked through desolation
to share His fellowship.
Doubt. I wept through despair to seek His faith.
Fear. I wrestled through darkness
to seize His freedom.

And the Balm of Gilead flowed
into the depths of my soul.
It cleansed; it soothed; it healed.

Again I cried, "Lord, use me!"
This time He answered, "Go!"
"I send you forth to heal.
Walk with the lonely.
Share with them My fellowship.
Weep with the despairing.
Seek with them My faith.
Wrestle with the fearful.
Seize with them My freedom.

And the Balm of Gilead will flow
into the depths of their souls.
It will cleanse;
It will soothe;
It will heal."

He spoke again: "My child,
I spared you no hurt—
that I might use you to heal."

~Peggie C. Bohanon

My Family Is Wondering

"When His family heard about this, they went to take charge of Him, for they said, 'He is out of His mind,'" (Mark 3:21).

The pain is real. Its severity varies from day to day, but it never diminishes. I could write a list of over two hundred descriptive words for the pain and still have more to add tomorrow. The pain is unlike anything I ever imagined. It is also invisible.

Family members ask me over the telephone how I am feeling. I try to answer both positively and honestly—no small feat. My common truthful answer is, "The body is falling apart, but the spirit is good." As we see one another in person, however, I am aware of their skeptical looks. Many of you have heard families whisper from the other room, "Do you really think he's in that much pain, or does he just not want to work?" You see how they analyze your moves when you carry a dish to the table but are unable to carry a glass a moment later. Do you feel like they think you're crazy?

Living with pain that is invisible is more of an emotional battle than physical. I adapt to pain, and I learn to be flexible in my plans. Even the stares when I park in a disabled spot are difficult to cope with, but these people are strangers and are not expected to understand. When my family, however, doubts the existence of my illness, it eats away at me, and I feel frustrated and betrayed.

Lord, they aren't sure what to believe about my condition. Some may believe that I am making the pain up for attention or sympathy. Give me the wisdom to be discerning in my words of reply when their words of skeptism are spoken. Let the truth shine through and my illness be acknowleged. Continue to be my source of strength when those closest to me disappoint me. Help me continue to love each of them the way that You intended, celebrating our relationship. *~Lisa Copen*

Learning To Be

"Now all has been heard; here is the conclusion of the matter: Fear God and keep His commandments, for this is the whole duty of man," (Ecclesiastes 12:13).

I recently drove from Virginia Beach to Richmond to attend the funeral service of a high school classmate. I graduated from high school in 1960, but many in my class have remained close, and we were together for the service. While traveling, my mind drifted back to those years in elementary and high school and the many dreams we all had for our lives. How many of us were successful? By whose standards?

Those of us suffering with chronic pain may feel anxious about the future. When we stop and consider what is really important, however, it is not about how many activities we are involved in, but our relationship with Jesus Christ. God is far more interested in a love relationship with us than He is interested in what we can do for Him. His desire is for us to love Him. When we follow God's leadership one day at a time, we will always be right in the middle of God's will for our lives. This is success by God's standards. This success is not measured by the world's standard for success. Even when the Lord tries to reassure us, Satan captures our thoughts, making us refuse to accept God's comfort. "When I was in distress, I sought the Lord; at night I stretched out untiring hands and my soul refused to be comforted," (Psalm 77:2). *Dear Jesus, give us a pure heart, that we may see Thee; a humble heart, that we may hear Thee; a heart of love, that we may serve Thee; a heart of faith, that we may live as Thee.*

Lord, don't let me worry about anything but pray about everything; thank You for Your answers. I want to experience Your peace, which is far more wonderful than the human mind can understand. "His peace will keep your thoughts and your hearts quiet… " (Philippians 4:6-7). *~Patricia Armstrong*

High Gear Or Low Gear?

"Before I was afflicted I went astray, but now I obey Your Word. It was good for me to be afflicted so that I might learn Your decrees," (Psalm 119:67,71).

With the fourth minor hurricane of the season behind us, I went out to ride my bike after a four day layoff from biking. It was hard to make myself ride, but I knew the end result would be in my favor. As I was riding along a back street, I shifted to a lower gear, which meant pedaling fewer times but pushing the pedals a little harder. I prefer the higher gears; it is easier to push the pedals, but then I have to pedal faster. Changing gears reminded me of some of the issues in living our lives with chronic pain.

Sometimes, we have to go slower, but it seems like more effort than what is required by living a faster pace. We can "coast" by some very important life issues when we run in higher gear. Being slowed down with daily chronic pain can help us to appreciate life's scenery. A slower pace affords us more time to be in God's Word, if we make the effort.

It takes great mental effort to live at a slower pace because we don't often have that momentum of everyday routine. Our days are often moments of "ups and downs," good days/not-so-good days. Yet we can greatly benefit from the extra effort, in the long run. For just as mild exercise oxygenates our bodies and helps them produce more energy during the metabolization process, the slowing down of our pace of life may also energize us, if we so choose.

Lord, help me to set goals that bring glory to You, and let me forget about the goals of this world. I want to live with no regrets! Only through You will I be able to find the right pace for this life and living with this illness. ~Ellie O'Steen

Transformation

"And we, who with unveiled faces all reflect the Lord's glory, are being transformed into His likeness with ever-increasing glory, which comes from the Lord, who is the Spirit,"(2 Corinthians 3:18).

God already knows what today holds for you. He knows if you will bump into someone who needs your friendly smile at the grocery store. He knows if you will get an email from someone who asks for prayer. God knows if you will stub your toe and cry out in pain or if you will sit on the couch and simply cry. He knows. He cares. He loves you.

You have a chronic illness. So do I. A thorn called rheumatoid arthritis burst into my life in 1993. Since medical science said, "It's chronic," that left me with just one alternative—healing. And yet, as much as I believed healing was possible, I didn't feel at peace about praying for it. I felt God calling me to use the thorn to glorify Him. I challenged God to do something more than just heal me. I wanted to be used.

We can't change our circumstances. Most of us may pray for healing, and yet in our hearts, we know that we will likely still wake up and not be healed tomorrow. This isn't a lack of faith; rather, it is the peace of our Lord saying, "My grace is sufficient." Circumstances will remain the same; however, we change. With every morning that we wake up and we are not healed, we are transformed a little more closely to his likeness. Jesus suffered. To be like Him, we must understand "the gift of pain," but the gift isn't a big empty box. It is not a white-elephant gift. We are being transformed into something *glorious*! Imagine it.

God, You know exactly what my day will hold today. My heart aches and depression abounds, even when I fight it. I can't change my circumstances, but I can hope in You, O Lord, because through this experience, You are creating something glorious—me!

~Lisa Copen

Uncomfortable Comforters

"I have called you friends, for everything that I learned from my Father I have made known to you," (John 15:15b).

Like peering in a mirror, the words of the young woman's testimony reflected my own pain and weakness. As she spoke, I recognized Nancy as a fellow soldier in the daily battle of living with chronic illness.

During the lunch break, Nancy and I discussed the challenges of chronic illness. Although suffering from different illnesses, we enjoyed the refreshing fellowship of sharing with someone who is traveling the same treacherous path. I left our time together heartened and with renewed strength.

According to John Henry Jowett, "God does not comfort us to make us comfortable, but to make us comforters."[33] As we receive encouragement from God, we have the joy and the responsibility to turn around and channel God's comfort to a fellow sufferer. At one time I thought I had to be completely well and comfortable before I could encourage those in hurting places. Self-centered in my own pain, I resisted opportunities to console others who were experiencing similar difficulties.

Patiently, God has shown me that I don't have to draw from some shallow well of comfort within myself in order to ease the suffering of another. He, "the God of all comfort," supplies an abundance of comfort. He eases my own pain and allows me to come alongside someone in distress.

God, through my chronic illness I have been given a unique ministry. Help me to reach out to the hurting by offering a listening ear and conversation that counts. I want to be able to offer Your balm, Lord, to those who are hurting. Bring people into my life who need Your healing salve, and give me the wisdom to know how to lift them up to You, Lord. *~Judy Gann*

My Body Is So Worn Out

"If you have raced with men on foot and they have worn you out, how can you compete with horses?" (Jeremiah 12:5b).

I have a precious baby doll named "Cindy," that I have had since I was five years old. Her hair is falling out, and what is left is matted. Her eyelashes are missing, and her cloth body has been repaired numerous times where the stuffing has fallen out. Some may look at her and think she has been abused; I look at her and see she has been loved.

How many times do we feel like an old doll? We may feel like the "stuffing" —our inner nature—is coming apart, and we feel lost, scared, and abandoned. We long for someone to recognize us for who we are, pick us up, care for us, and sympathize with our needs. Our outward appearance does not reflect the inner person that is crying to be loved like the "velveteen rabbit."

"I have upheld you since you were conceived, and carried you since your birth. Even to your old age and gray hairs, I am He who will sustain you. I have made you, and I will carry you, and I will rescue you," (Isaiah 46:3,4). Place your hope and trust in God, and He will meet your needs. He will transform your inner nature, spirit, and soul. He will walk beside you, hand in hand, through the pain and suffering you are going through. "The Lord will watch over your coming and going, both now and forevermore," (Psalm 121:8).

Cindy has been cleaned up and sits upon my hope chest in my bedroom. She wears a sweet infant dress, bonnet, tights, and shoes. She has never looked better, for she has become "real."

God, work in my life today and transform me into someone authentic who is purely Your child above all my other identities.

~Kay DeCarlo

The Road Of Life

The road of life leads many ways,
Some easy and some hard to bear.
But God has promised to stay by our side,
Our sufferings and heartaches to share.

Think back for a moment to Calvary's hill,
Where Jesus suffered alone.
He shed His lifeblood, He suffered the pain,
For everyone's sin to atone.

This task wasn't easy, but He went to the end,
Was victor o'er all of the test.
And now all He asks of you and of me,
Is that each of us give Him our best.

Sometimes there are hills that take us high,
Then, times there are valleys so low.
In times like these we can be sure,
God leads us as we go.

Some days are bright with God's great love,
Some days the sky looks dim.
But just press on, hold on to faith,
Put all your trust in Him.

He never fails; He's always there,
To bring sweet peace within.
If we will live a Christ-like life,
And turn away from sin.

He gives us strength to overcome,
Grace to help endure.
God's love and presence is with you,
Of this you can be sure.

So yield to God, give Him your all,
Give Him your very best.
If we will pray and do our part,
God will take care of the rest.

~Ada Mahle

I Need A Good Cry

"He will wipe every tear from their eyes. There will be no more death or mourning or crying or pain, for the old order of things has passed away," (Revelation 21:4).

I recently heard the saying, "I always knew that looking back at my tears would make me laugh, but I never thought that looking back at my laughter would make me cry." It can be hard to grieve, but have you wondered if a good cry wouldn't be rejuvenating? A few months have passed since one of those "I-just-can't-take-this-another-minute!" moments. I've taken things one day at a time, pushing my feelings aside. Sometimes, this *can* be a good thing. If we spent all of our time dwelling and crying over every ailment, we'd never leave our bedroom, and we'd be advised by family members to buy stock in Kleenex®. Still, a good cry can shed those piled-up emotions, the frustrations, even the desperation. Regardless of whether we cuddle up in a loved one's arms to shed our sorrows or stand alone in the shower and let the tears flow over us with the water, we never, ever cry alone.

Even David felt overwhelmed and frustrated, and he cried. "My tears have been my food day and night, while men say to me all day long, 'Where is your God?'" (Psalms 42:3). He felt like God had abandoned him, but God was there, looking over him especially while he was in tears.

Psalm 56:8 says that God gathers up our tears and stores them in a wineskin. He records them on His scroll. He knows about every tear we shed, and they are precious to Him. He too has cried tears when He was overwhelmed at the pain and sin in the world (John 11:35). He understands. He also promises that there will be no tears in heaven.

Revelation 21:4 says, "[You] will wipe every tear from [my] eyes. There will be no more death or mourning or crying or pain, for the old order of things has passed away." Lord, I won't need any hankies in heaven.

~Lisa Copen

The Goodness of Yesterday and Today

"This is because both of you broke faith with Me in the presence of the Israelites, at the waters of Meribah Kadesh, in the Desert of Zion, and because you did not uphold My holiness among the Israelites," (Deuteronomy 32:51).

My heart goes out to Moses. We think of him as a superhero that overcame all obstacles to free his people and lead them to the Promised Land. Even so, his mistake of hitting the rock instead of speaking to it, as God directed, meant that he was not allowed to enter the Promised Land. Bottom line, the Israelites were whining and complaining, having forgotten the provision of God. It is like saying, "Well, the miracles of yesterday were great, but what have you done for me today?" Moses lost his temper with his people and smacked the rock. God gave them water anyway, and Moses was welcomed to heaven because God is good and merciful. It is comforting to know that God loves us even when we mess up.

Many days, I am a great deal like Moses. *Yes, Lord, the goodness of yesterday was great, but how about today?* I am still in pain; I am unable to do all that I wish; my circumstances have not changed. Okay, so we had sunshine yesterday, and I am warm and dry. Yes, my stomach is full, and I have a loving family. Oh look, the roses are blooming, and I can go out and smell them. Provision is here, goodness abounds, but I always find reasons to want something else. We lack freedom. However, Luke 6:25 in *The Message* reminds us, "There's trouble ahead if you're satisfied with yourself. Yourself will not satisfy you for long."

Lord God, I want what I cannot have, and I can't always see what I do have. It is a good thing I am not in control; I am fortunate You are in control and that You love me no matter what. I am here for a reason. Today exists – for me. Lord, give me strength and direction for my calling. Lead me. ~*Rebecca Koszalinski*

A Thread Of Hope

"...We who have fled to take hold of the hope offered to us may be greatly encouraged. We have the hope as an anchor for the soul, firm and secure," (Hebrews 6:18-19).

Sprawled out in bed today, trying to focus on something other than the pain, my eyes are fixed on an old patchwork quilt that my grandmother made decades ago. She used a wide variety of clothes, all of different textures and colors, hand-sewn together to construct this unique spread.

Through the years, however, age and stress have made the fabrics vulnerable to tattering. Thousands of strings that were once tightly knitted together to form a lovely blanket, are now exposing loose threads that, if pulled, could possibly unravel the entire piece of fabric.

This quilt is a good example of people with chronic illness. We are bonded together by the painful circumstances of our lives, yet are otherwise individual and unique. The pain, depression, and frustration that chronic illness places in our lives, can leave us feeling weak and vulnerable, as though we have loose threads just waiting to come unraveled. Corrie ten Boom says, "It is good to regret missed opportunities, but quite wrong to be miserable without them."[34]

The book of Hebrews reminds us today that, when we feel despair, there is a thread of hope that we can hold on to. This hope is found with our Lord, Jesus Christ, and promises to be firm and secure. Do you feel as though the pain, frustration, and depression in your life is causing you to unravel? Hang on today, dear child. Don't let go of that thread of hope.

Lord, Your threads are secure and will pull me through. Help me tie a knot and hang on for this experience, but never let the threads break. I need You, O Lord, how I need You. *~Deborah Farmer*

Learning Through Depression

"Cursed is the man who trusts in man and makes flesh his strength, whose heart departs from the Lord," (Jeremiah 17:5).

My circumstances are unique because I went through a three-year period of depression *before* I was diagnosed with fibromyalgia or myofascial pain syndrome. God taught me a lot about myself and about Him. Once, I had believed that I needed to be in control of myself and other people because of my issues with insecurity and significance. I knew in my heart I should deal with these things, but I ignored them. God wanted me to deal with them.

He allowed my hormones to go haywire when I was experiencing other life and relational changes. I now had no illusion that I was in control, and a black cloud of depression settled over my life. I was no longer emotionally strong enough to suppress or ignore my heart. My joy left, and I wrote in my journal, "Lord, wash away this fear that dominates me. Give me the grace to freely love again."

In *The Storm Within* author Mark Littleton writes: "If you are severely depressed and wading through the murk of inexplicable suffering, keep this one thought in mind: God can and will use this for good in [my] life. He will teach [me] patience and goodness and a hope that can never be broken.' Tell yourself this over and over… You won't believe it at times. You will hate the idea and, at times, the author of it. Your mind will rationalize it, argue against it, shout you down. But be steadfast and believe it. God is working. He will not waste even this. He will redeem it and out of it bring benefits that you will rejoice to see."[35] My prayers began to change.

Lord, redirect me. Give my life the meaning You always wanted it to be in service and worship to You. I want more of You. Lord, please use the things I've been through to bring others hope.

~Sheryl Smith

I Can't Put Life On Hold

"I wait for the Lord, my soul waits, and in His Word I put my hope," (Psalms 130:5).

Sometimes I wonder if doctors take pleasure in having their patients wait for them. Don't we all wish someone would wait to see us? They often have very tight schedules, but have you ever wondered if they believe patients will respect them more if we must wait for the privilege of speaking to them? Does waiting cause us to be more submissive? Does time break down our memory, causing us to forget the questions that we were going to ask? Regardless, we spend much of our time waiting for life to start. Like John Lennon said, "Life is what happens when you are making other plans."

We can't slow time down. When we live with constant pain, it can be hard to avoid the mindset of, "When I feel better I will…" do this or that. Depending on my current flare level, I may decide to participate in something or skip it. For example, when the county fair arrives, if I think I can walk a little, I want to go. It's pointless to compare it to former days when I could walk around for twelve hours, eat whatever I wanted, and go on a few rides. Those days are over. Now I have the choice to go for a few hours, and I may even use a wheelchair. I can be sad or mad about it, or I can just go and make the best of it and create some new memories. The old adage "Time heals all wounds" is not true for those with chronic illness. Time may pass, but the illness stays.

Before I was diagnosed, I thought a drug would quickly get me back to normal. After diagnosis, the doctors sounded positive, and they prescribed all kinds of medications to get me into remission and then wean me off the drugs. I never got to remission. They continued to raise the dosages and add new medications.

God, don't let me wait to be well. Help me wait for You to do what You are going to do while I put my hope in You. ~*Lisa Copen*

I Carry A Burden

"Come to Me, all you who are weary and burdened, and I will give you rest. Take My yoke upon you and learn from Me, for I am gentle and humble in heart, and you will find rest for your souls," (Matthew 11:28,29).

I carry a burden not easily seen and which most people my age don't understand. My burden is stacked several boxes high, and I must carefully balance it, or it will crash down on me, hurting me more severely than usual.

My burden is heavy, and it causes me pain, but the worst part of it is the lack of freedom. I can't use my body for other things, so consumed am I by carrying this burden.

I walk down the path of my life, and I see all around me other people walking their paths, only they walk so freely and confidently while I labor on with my load.

Sometimes I think about my former self, the me before this burden was imposed. I wasn't perfect by any means, but I could escape from my troubles. And now there is no escape, never an escape; not for ten years has there been an escape. My burden is always there, even when I sleep. And I can't take a vacation from it.

In the early days and months, people were concerned, and they offered to help me carry my stack. They walked next to me as I struggled along, lightening my arms just a little.

More recently people don't draw near so much, and I struggle with painful loneliness. I struggle with painful isolation, and I question my worth if people can leave me like this.

It's not that other people don't care about me; they're just too busy with their own cares. If I could go out into their world, their lives, I probably wouldn't feel so alone, but my whole world exists here at home.

I want to take my burden off. I want to stand on a cliff and hurl it out into the sea. I want to have my body back. To dance, to run, to jump, to sit or stand without counting the

(continued)

minutes. I've tried every way you can imagine to throw off this weight of limitations, and I have to face my own powerlessness at failing to do so.

Or, if I can't get rid of my burden, I want, in my blackest heart of hearts, to burden everyone else with the same limitations. I want to see how well others would cope, and I want to make them know how difficult my life is and punish them for being indifferent to me.

Just please don't flaunt your lack of burdens to me. It cuts me so deeply to know you are free. Please don't tell me about your vacations; your sports; your second incomes and wonderful careers; your new homes; your great weekends; your second, third, and fourth children, which I can't have. . . You see, I'm dying inside when I hear these things.

Please don't look at me in shock when I say I can't sit long enough for a movie or meet you for lunch. Don't look at me like I'm odd when I have to lie down. Don't tell me, "I could never live like you have to," because I can't do this either! Do you think this is all okay with me?

I guess that's why I'm seeking out others who carry great burdens, so we can learn together how to survive. You high achievers can go on ahead. There are things we're learning that you just can't understand. I used to be just like you, full of my own strength and promise and success, but I'm finding there are lessons in brokenness that deepen a person as success cannot.

My life experience used to be about two miles wide and one foot in depth. Now my life experience is about two feet wide and a mile in depth. It contains the same volume, but it's so much deeper. The roots sunk so much more securely in God's promises than in my own promise.

My own promise feels like a joke to me now; it can be ripped away and shredded up and spit out. But God's promises can't be ripped, shredded, or spit. They are for *real.* "The heavens and earth may pass away, but My Word will never pass away," (Luke 21:33).

Still, it's painful to be pruned. It's hard to be melted

(continued)

so the impurities come out. The process threatens to dump me into despair, and I must cling to my faith that God's hand is in this; I'm His pot, His clay, and He's forming me. I didn't want to hurt this much.

I didn't want to be a plain pot, such a humble pot, but one that people admired and that accomplished a lot; the kind of pot that I defined as "successful." But I can choose to accept that I'm the clay pot He wants; if I don't belong to myself, I belong to Him. And it's His decision how I am shaped and fired and glazed, even though my ideas looked better to me.

And a pot I designed would have fit more comfortably than this rougher, harder, more awkward-fitting pot I have. The pot I wanted was always in use at great parties, with people all around. The pot that I am is often hidden away in a dark closet and briefly exposed to the light or to people, but mostly kept quiet and away from the excitement of life. And for reasons only God knows, that is where I belong.

But such a pot, when chosen, knows it is not for superficial reasons, but for real qualities. Such a pot has a real spirit of humility because its ego is broken. Such a pot can be at peace, knowing it doesn't have to seek after purposes and uses. But its Maker will call it into service when ready. Such a pot learns to submit, to surrender, to rest in its Maker's loving arms.

Lord, I want to be that beautiful pot that You desire me to be, but the process is so painful. Give me the daily affirmation that You are always beside me and that nothing in this world will happen to me that has not been Your intention.

~Roxanne M. Smith

All Lemonade Isn't Sour

"Therefore encourage one another and build each other up... And we urge you, brothers, warn those who are idle, encourage the timid, help the weak, be patient with everyone," (1 Thessalonians 5:11a,14).

A very wise and dear friend of mine once gave me good advice. While I was struggling with my diagnosis of rheumatoid arthritis, my friend sent me a floral arrangement, decorated around a lemon squeezer. Attached to the squeezer was the message, "When life gives you a bunch of lemons, make lemonade!" At that time, I had two choices: I could pucker up and become a miserable sourpuss, or I could accept my circumstances and adhere to my friend's advice. I chose to make lemonade! Those lemons became faith builders rather than destroyers.

I thank God my friend took the time to encourage me, in a unique and fun-loving way, to "make lemonade." I experienced the greatest spiritual growth of my life at that time because this friend cared enough to reach out to me in Christian love and concern; my hope, trust, and faith in a loving God were restored and strengthened!

C.S. Lewis wrote in *The Problem of Pain:* "Pain is not good in itself. What is good in any painful experience is, for the sufferer, his submission to the will of God, and, for the spectators, the compassion aroused and the acts of mercy to which it leads."[36] Dear friends, I urge you to get into the business of faith-building. Because of my friend, "I am greatly encouraged; in all [my] troubles my joy knows no bounds," (2 Corinthians 7:4).

Lord, teach me how to dig deeply into Your Word, to search for Your answers and encouragement. Teach me to reach out to others and learn to accept the encouragement people give me with joy.

~Nancy Wilcox

We Will See Him In The Pain

"There they will see Me," (Matthew 28:10).

This was the second time that Jesus told His disciples that they would see Him in Galilee. Jesus never tires of telling us something over and over again; He patiently teaches us as many times as it takes for us to understand.

There they would see Him. And it is here that we will see Him, in this chronic illness. For this might be the only set of circumstances in which we see His faithfulness, His comfort, His tenderness, or His love. Although I want nothing more than for the pain or the fatigue to go away, His desire is for me to see Him and share intimate fellowship with Him. For some of us, this might be the only way for that to happen. It does not stop there, for after we "see" Him, then He tells us to "go and tell my brethren" what He is like.

We are not to keep Him to ourselves! "Comfort, comfort my people, says your God," (Isaiah 40:1). We are to let what we see of Him pass through us, and then reach out to others, so that they might see and experience Him also and know of His love, tenderness, comfort, and faithfulness. Paul's greatest ministry occurred while He sat in prison in chains. Jesus knew He had only three years to reach the multitudes with the Truth. Our illness is our tool, not our deterrent.

Let God open your eyes, dear one, so that you might see Him and His tender love through you. Many people with illness and weakness are living examples of how God provides for all one's needs within the pain.

Please open my eyes, Lord. Help me see You, even in the pain. Teach me how to find the treasures in the darkness, the gifts in the pain. I want to know You, Lord. Open my eyes.

~Virginia Ganskie

Picking Up The Prayer Line

"'Call to me and I will answer you and tell you great and unsearchable things you do not know,'" (Jeremiah 33:3).

When the phone rings, I make a choice to answer it or to let the machine take a message. Isn't it a wonder how technology has led us to forget how to be personal with our friends and loved ones? It can be difficult to keep in close contact with one another because everyone is in a rush to get to their jobs, do errands, or run off to events. Sometimes, we just do not want to pick up the phone, and we let the machine take the place of us.

I'm not saying that technology hasn't helped us. It has, but sometimes I think we go too far and become lazy. That's how I was feeling a few days ago. I was not in a good mood or feeling well when the phone rang, and it was a sister in Christ, calling to pray and encourage me. I let the machine take a message, and I missed out on a real blessing from God.

Sometimes, we are like this with the Lord God; we back off and miss out on His blessings. Instead of listening for God's message in our innermost being, we let our moods or circumstances get the best of us; we "let the machine get God's message," and we never even hear it. God knows our every need, and He is always on time for us. When He is speaking to us, we must be ready to listen. We must keep our prayer line open and make contact to receive from the Almighty God. By seeking Him in prayer, His Word, or through our brothers and sisters in Christ, we can hear God.

"Let us not give up meeting together, as some are in the habit of doing, but let us encourage one another and all the more as you see the day approaching," (Hebrews 10:25). Lord, help me to keep the prayer line open; don't let my line be broken.

~ Mary Ann Redondo

What Glasses Do You Wear?

"Now we see but a poor reflection as in a mirror; then we shall see face to face. Now I know in part; then I shall know fully, even as I am fully known," (1 Corinthians 13:12).

I've had many eye problems during the past year but have finally received new glasses, stabilizing my vision. During this time, I have been able to see through spiritual eyes. Bible verses and promises from Scripture, that I learned as a child in Sunday School, came back to me. Through His grace and tender mercy, the Lord has prompted me to "see" exactly what He wanted me to envision. Through another limitation, He has taught me patience and trust. He has increased my faith.

Each of us wears some kind of glasses—if not real ones, then imaginary ones. Every so often we see life through "gray lenses," seeing only gloom and doom. On these days we are actually shutting God out of our lives. On another day, we might wear "rose-colored glasses" and easily be misled by what we see and hear. Or, we might intentionally put on our "cloudy glasses" to escape the realities of living with chronic conditions.

Hopefully, we have many days when we wear "clear lenses." When we wear clear lenses, we are better able to find God and trust in Him even though we don't understand our situation or why we must live with chronic illness. Paradoxically, our vision becomes the clearest at the point when we willingly walk by faith and not by sight. Our "trust walk" liberates us as we rely on the Lord and not upon ourselves.

I will trust in You, Lord, with all my heart, and lean not on my own understanding; in all my ways I acknowledge You, and You will make my paths straight. Do not allow me to be wise in my own eyes; help me fear You and shun evil, (Proverbs 3:6-7, paraphrased).

~Nancy Wilcox

Turning Toward Those Who Care

"Because He turned His ear to me, I will call on Him as long as I live," (Psalm 116:1,2).

In 1860, Florence Nightingale wrote the following in *Notes on Nursing: What It Is and What It Is Not:* "It is a curious thing to observe how almost all patients lie with their faces turned to the light, exactly as plants always make their way towards the light; a patient will even complain that it gives him pain 'lying on that side.' 'Then why do you lie on that side?' He does not know, but we do. . . ."[37]

When I was diagnosed with my illness, it was an interesting, and sometimes heartbreaking experience to observe which friends would stick around and who would fade away. At the time, I was involved and working part-time at a church that was more interested in my healing than my heart. A few coworkers did their best to offer kindness, but I felt the stares of the power-suited women who glanced at my ugly but necessary shoes. "I know just how you feel," some would bellow. "I worked out last night at the gym." More tears were shed because of my sensitivity to words, than my new requirement of a higher tolerance of pain.

I prayed for a friend to accompany me on the journey, a "sister in pain" who could keep me laughing over my illness so I wouldn't cry. God sent me Connie. From the moment she called to ask me for coffee, I felt a kinship. She too defied advice about drinking caffeine and was a sister in Christ. The light of a friend is sometimes all we need to bring us back to a place where we can hear God again.

Psalm 68:6 says, "God sets the lonely in families." God, bring me family within this new life that includes disease. I pray for a friend, for a mentor. I ask for someone with whom I can laugh with, cry with, and who will understand the mixed emotions of joy and pain. Friendship is not about being perfect, it is just about being there. I need someone here, Lord. ~*Lisa Copen*

The Shepherd's Oil

"You prepare a table before me in the presence of my enemies. You anoint my head with oil; my cup overflows," (Psalm 23:5).

When David wrote the twenty-third Psalm, it was believed that his son Absalom had already forcibly seized the throne and had exiled David from Jerusalem. David had lost his throne, crown, authority, scepter, followers, and his kingdom. He had lost nearly all of his worldly possessions; yet he writes, "The Lord is my Shepherd. I shall not want." God is a loving Shepherd. We, the Lord's sheep, can look to our Shepherd for protection, leadership, and guidance when we are facing evil and suffering. God shows His loving kindness and protecting power to us.

Oil was used for anointing. Jesus was named the Anointed One. When David was proclaimed as king, head was anointed with oil. David refers to the Lord as the Heavenly Shepherd, one who is anointing His children with oil, thus giving us a royal place in His kingdom. This reminds us that we are loved by a Shepherd who wants to bestow His grace on us today. Oil was also used as a soothing balm; the Shepherd would rub oil on the wounds of the sheep to clean and promote healing. Sometimes a sheep would wander into a path of danger, and the shepherd would search for the lost lamb, tending to its individual needs.

Do you have deep wounds today? Bruises that this cruel world has given you? Deep cuts from pain, death, or depression? Painful gashes from illness or isolation? Draw close to the Heavenly Shepherd. "[One] intended it to harm me, but God intended it for good to accomplish what is now being done, the saving of many lives," (Genesis 50:20).

Lord, You desire to anoint me with Your oil. As Shepherd, You may not change the bad times, but You will not abandon me. You will soothe these wounds and hold me close to You so I can endure the trial, and find rest and comfort. *~Deborah Farmer*

Pushing Beyond Our Ability

"For I testify that they gave as much as they were able, and even beyond their ability," (2 Corinthians 8:3).

I laugh at myself as I quickly answer the ringing phone and, in an exasperated voice, say, "Rest Ministries!" Rest. It is something that we must redefine when we become chronically ill. I recently saw a book chapter entitled *Recognizing Burnout Before You're Charred.* How often we push ourselves until we become charred. Not only do we do as much as we are able, but we also push farther past our abilities. It takes all of our energy to accomplish the basics, such as showering and dressing; every task becomes more time consuming. In the past couple of weeks, my prayer has been, "Lord, multiply my time and my strength."

There are days that you will do much that is beyond your ability—the day your daughter turns thirteen and you have a slumber party for seven girls; the day that your parents celebrate their fiftieth wedding anniversary and your siblings leave the organizing to you since you live the closest. Perhaps you will give beyond your ability during difficult times—when you father goes into the nursing home or your best friend tells you that she has cancer.

There is no denying that moments will arise when we must put our illness aside and push forward. We push through the pain and exhaustion so we can participate in necessary moments of life. If you read the previous verse, 2 Corinthians 8:2, it explains the irony of why we give beyond our ability. "Out of the most severe trial, their overflowing joy and their extreme poverty welled up in rich generosity."

God, it is no secret that I will experience that extreme poverty, but I will also experience overflowing joy, and out of both of these circumstances, I will end up with a desire to give to others—even when it involves giving beyond my ability. ~Lisa Copen

The Wonders Of Him

"I have learned the secret of being content in any and every situation," (Philippians 4:12b).

I was born with a disorder called neurofibromatosis, and it causes many health problems; it is often disfiguring. Lately, my disorder has become worse. This has brought me to my knees in prayer, worship, and the study of God's Word.

In the midst of this, I have found myself seeking the Lord God through prayer, praise, and reading His Word. This has helped me to walk through the trials and circumstances, which accompany my pain. There were times I could not pick up the Bible but just would sit and talk with the Lord about how I was feeling, and what came to my remembrance was how Moses, King David, Paul, John, and Jesus Himself coped when they were faced with trials. God spoke to them when they found the quiet time to be still in Him. When I decided to do this, to find my quiet time with The Lord; what happened next was a peace that washed over me and engulfed me. My pain was still there, but His words whispered within me, "My grace is sufficient for you, for My power is made perfect in weakness," (2 Corinthians 12:9). His words also reminded me, "He will never leave me nor forsake me," (Deuteronomy 31:6). For I know who holds my future no matter what comes my way!

My relationship with the Lord God has grown, and I enjoy our times together each day. When I am distressed with pain, I run to my Strong Tower of Refuge. The Lord is my strong tower; He lifts me up with His comfort that surpasses all understanding. "The name of the Lord is a strong tower; the righteous run to it and they are safe," (Proverbs 18:10).

You say You will, "strengthen the feeble hands, steady the knees that give way," (Isaiah 35:3). "When He spoke to me, I was strengthened," (Daniel 10:19). Speak to me, Lord. I am listening.

~Mary Ann Redondo

I Want To Be A Mom

"I prayed for this child, and the Lord has granted me what I asked of Him," (1 Samuel 1:27).

We've been waiting for a child for years—most recently, over two years to adopt. Someone said having a child was one of the most selfish things I could do. "How are you going to care for it? What kinds of opportunities will the child have?"

Long before we began to consider having a child, I asked myself these same questions. My husband and I had many conversations about our life with a child. I read books. I spoke with other women who had chronic illnesses and listened to their experiences. And I came to the conclusion that, despite this illness, I am going to be a fabulous (and humble?) parent. There will be times I will wonder, *What have I gotten myself into?* But what parent doesn't have those worries? I understand that parenting will be the hardest task I will take on, but I'm not going to let my illness take away the joy that I can experience by being a mom. Jesus's parents lost track of Him for three days before they even realized that He was missing. Surely, I can be at least that efficient!

Whether your desire is to have a child or not have a child, search for God's desire for your life. Do not pay attention to the cruel comments, the twisted advice, or the looks of doubt you may receive from others. Every family adapts to its strengths and weaknesses. God carefully plans the family in which you will reside. Although illness may alter many of our own plans, illnesses never alter God's plans for our lives. He always knew the challenges we would face, and He has been preparing us, in His perfect way, for His perfect timing. I know it's all true, but yes, I understand just how hard it is to wait. It's something I must surrender daily.

"In the morning, O Lord, You hear my voice; in the morning, I lay my requests before You and wait in expectation," (Psalm 5:3).

~Lisa Copen

Weaknesses Play A Part

"That is why for Christ's sake, I delight in weaknesses, in insults, in hardships, in persecutions, in difficulties," (2 Corinthians 12:10).

Oftentimes, before I leave the grocery store, I ask a clerk to open up a jar that contains an ingredient for that evening's meal. Despite the fact that we can send a man to outer space, we are unable to design an effective jar opener. At one time, I dreaded asking for help. I would plan my exact words as the clerk tallied my bill. Then I would blurt out, "Please open this jar. . . I have rheumatoid arthritis,"so quickly that he would have to ask me to repeat myself. As the clerk would pop the jar open, embarrassment would seep through me, frustrated that he realized, or even doubted, my weakness.

Over time, I have learned to accept that it is better to reveal my weakness and ask for help than to spend twenty frustrating minutes trying to open a jar, only to end up with spaghetti sauce laced with broken glass. With my admission of weakness, however, has come an opportunity to share a very personal part of my life. I don't corner anyone to tell them about God, but I do explain I have an illness, and when they ask questions, I tell them about my ministry for the chronically ill. Who am I to guess how the Holy Spirit works? By asking a clerk to open up my bottled water, could I be planting a seed to lead him to Christ? Regardless, God is magnified because of my weakness.

Once, I believed that it would be my strengths that would best serve God, but in time I am learning it is through my weaknesses that He is most glorified. 2 Corinthians 12:10 says, "That is why, for Christ's sake, I delight in weaknesses. . . . in difficulties. For when I am weak, then I am strong."

Before recently, Lord, I didn't understand the business about delighting in my weaknesses. Day by day, I am beginning to find delight in seeing what You are going to do with my next limitation. I have lots of weaknesses for You to choose from. ~*Lisa Copen*

I Am Worried

"Who of you can add a single hour to his life by worrying? Since you cannot do this very little thing, why do you worry about the rest?" (Luke 12:25,26).

The United States Public Health Service recently issued a statement presenting statistics about how one's habit to worry can shorten one's life. Still, I've spent the last few days anxiously awaiting test results; I don't want them to be positive, but if they are negative, it will only mean another series of tests and a continued lack of diagnosis. I can't help it; I'm worried.

Worry doesn't do any good. I logically know this to be true, but sometimes it is hard to put God's Word into practice in my daily life. Jesus asks, "Who of you can add a single hour to his life by worrying? Since you cannot do this very little thing, why do you worry about the rest?" (Luke 12:25,26). He had a point. I think my worries have taken a few days off of my life! Through these verses, Jesus is emphasizing our lack of control in our life. I certainly feel this lack of control today. As much as I try, I can't will the phone to ring or have the test results be negative. He is, however, affirming that although I lack control, He does not. Attitude is important. I can choose to worry, or I can choose to surrender my worries over to Him and go about my day.

Corrie ten Boom once wrote, "Worry does not empty tomorrow of its sorrows; it empties today of its strength."[38] Worries often multiply when there is nothing around to distract one from them. In the past, I have turned to my Bible, called a friend or taken a drive and slipped some fun music in the stereo. I have to turn it over to God.

Lord, I need to provide a consistent home for trust and peace to reside, and leave worry outside the door. Life is too short to worry about what may happen. Help me "encourage one another daily," (Hebrews 3:13). *~Lisa Copen*

I Will Not Be Consumed

"Because of the Lord's great love we are not consumed, for His compassions never fail. They are new every morning; great is Your faithfulness. I say to myself, 'The Lord is my portion; therefore I will wait for Him,'" (Lamentations 3:22-24).

Someone recently asked me to share a verse that had gotten me through those difficult moments of coping with infertility and chronic illness. I explained that the verse above was the one that brought me comfort, but it also guarded my heart and brought me hope for what God has planned. Diagnosed with a chronic illness ten years earlier, the first question I asked was, "Will I still be able to have children?" The answer was yes, and I clung to this hope that, despite all that this illness would take away, it would not take away my ability to be a mother. God had other plans....

Years later, I discovered that, due to medications, I would be unable to have children; I refused to become obsessive about the loss that threatened to break my spirit, as I had seen many women lose all sense of reality, hope, and even marriages in the grieving process. This verse I loved had even greater meaning. I would *not* be consumed because of God's love. God also realizes that, although I can momentarily convince myself of this, I need His renewal every twenty-four hours; I need specific assurance that His mercies are new every morning. God doesn't take weekends off.

My husband and I have been waiting to adopt a baby for a long time, and as I write this, we are still in the depths of expectantly waiting for that which we feel will make our family "its full portion." It's never easy. That's why we have to renew ourselves each morning in His Word and claim, "Lord, You are my full portion."

Lord, great is Thy faithfulness. You are my full portion – not just half. I will give You all my longings and cling to Your hope so I will not be consumed by all my earthly desires. *~Lisa Copen*

Suffering Unjustly

"For it is commendable if a man bears up under the pain of unjust suffering because he is conscious of God. To this you were called, because Christ suffered for you, leaving you an example, that you should follow in His steps," (1 Peter 2:18, 21).

Before I was diagnosed with an illness, I was a twenty-four-year-old girl who thought that anything was possible with enough motivation and persistence. I thrived on doing more than others expected, and the best compliment I could receive was, "I just don't know how you do it all." When I became ill, life changed, but my attitude didn't. I was determined that I would continue to live like I always had.

Despite my attitude, my life did change significantly: I prioritized—not just my activities, but my relationships, values, and my dreams. I had a hard outer shell, but I must admit, inside I was frightened. I had many sleepless nights, wondering what I would do when I could no longer control the outcome. None of us "deserve" our illness. It is my belief that God does not punish with illness for our sins.

Illness is simply a result of the sin of our world. However, He can use it for good. He does realize that it is unfair and that we long for those days when we could awake feeling refreshed, the days when we didn't know the pharmacists by their first names. However, "it is commendable if a man bears up under the pain of unjust suffering." Commendable means praiseworthy, admirable, worthy—but we are only these things because we are conscious of God.

Like many of the apostles, I am suffering. I may be walking the journey of chronic illness, yet I can take heart that Christ Himself has treaded down the grass of this pathway and "I should simply follow in His steps." Apostles have also worn the path down to soften the dirt, so my step is a bit easier, and Your angels have planted daisies along the way, all to make me more conscious of You.

~Lisa Copen

Interceding For You

"In the same way, the Spirit helps us in our weakness: We do not know what we ought to pray for, but the Spirit Himself intercedes for us with groans that words cannot express," (Romans 8:26).

The long dark nights are the hardest to endure when we are consumed with pain. Every dart of discomfort and every spark of hurt is magnified in the still quietness of the night. I seek rest yet cannot find it. I try to sleep, but pain forces me to suffer quietly, as my heart continues to grow more heavy and discouraged. Sometimes, I am still awake after the tears, and the minutes slowly tick away. It is during these moments that I cannot focus enough to pray elaborately; all I can do is groan. In Romans 8:26 Paul reminds us that our prayers are always heard. Even when all I can say to the Lord is "SOS!" I know that the Holy Spirit is interpreting my emotions and interceding to the Father on my behalf. We are blessed to have a loving Heavenly Father who knows the mind of our intercessor. We have the risen Christ at the right hand of the Father, interceding for us.

Intercession is having someone in a position of influence, pleading on our behalf. Jesus is that intercessor for us. Within the Trinity, where communication is perfectly expressed and perfectly understood above any level of communication we could ever comprehend, it is a comfort to know that we are being represented by One who also has suffered while He was here on earth and knows our pain intimately. So, even when our prayers seem awkward, laced with confusion, we can know that they are being presented to the Loving Father. He hears our hearts.

Lord, my prayers are heard, and I can trust You to use the pain in my life to strengthen me and prepare me for Your purpose. Knowing this can make that long dreary night more bearable. Lord, I am sending out my SOS to You, who are waiting to intercede on my behalf today. *~Deborah Farmer*

Gaining In Losing

"What is more, I consider everything a loss compared to the surpassing greatness of knowing Christ Jesus my Lord, for whose sake I have lost all things. I consider them rubbish, that I may gain Christ," (Philippians 3:8).

Loss is a daily part of life when one lives with a chronic illness. It occurs too frequently, as we discover that we have been diagnosed with another illness, a good friend divorces, or a pet must be put to sleep. Our mind no longer seems to work as clearly or efficiently as it once did. On the other hand, success seems to surround us—sometimes even mock us. Sitting at a stoplight a few days ago, I looked around to discover that I was the only one at the light with an actual license plate. Everyone else was driving a new vehicle. Friends boast that they are working "just for the fun of it." because they don't really need the money after their wise investments. Others' grocery carts are filled bountifully.

The rest of the world is gaining success, possessions, and status as we, who sit in the midst of our losses, are the ones who will have everlasting life. For everything that we may succeed in or gain, that is not Jesus Christ, is considered a loss, for when we believe in Christ, we have gained the only thing in life that is worth gaining. Illness may have zapped your spunk; the news from a doctor is disappointing; perhaps a friend let you down. But take heart because you have gained all that you need to gain in this world to get by. New cars, fancy clothes, the ticket stubs from the hot concert that you didn't get to attend—all are rubbish in this world. Illness filters out temptations in life; we long for comfort, not concerts. C.S. Lewis wrote, "The only people who achieve much, are those who want knowledge so badly, that they seek it while the conditions are still unfavorable. Favorable conditions never come."[39] We must change our attitude now.

Jesus, You will give me surpassing greatness. Help me seek it in the very depths of the darkness. ~*Lisa Copen*

The Darkest Season

"Be anxious for nothing, but in everything, by prayer and supplication, with thanksgiving, let your requests be made known to God; and the peace of God, which surpasses all understanding, will guard your hearts and minds through Christ Jesus," (Philippians 4:6-7).

Depression. What is it that makes us feel we can't possibly face another day? Where does this feeling of hopelessness come from? How do we move on? *Can* we move on?

There is a long-believed theory that all Christians experience a season of total darkness. The dark period is not a punishment, but one feels as though s/he will never feel God's presence again. Scripture seems uninspiring. No one seems to understand. We can't always find a reason for a lack of feeling God's presence; sometimes it just happens. However, God does pull one through it, and when one comes out on the other side of this seemingly endless, dark tunnel, one realizes the immense depth of his faith.

When there is no logical reason to have faith in God, continue to have it! This feeling of claiming your faith, even in the most desperate of circumstances, is a strong foundation for life. You may be feeling deep depression. Or you may not understand how "good Christians" can ever feel hopeless, but it is possible. It's not from lack of faith. It's a season.

The Bible says, "…the peace of God, which surpasses all understanding, will guard your hearts *and minds* through Christ Jesus," (Philippians 4:6-7; italics added). I believe that it's important we realize that our *thoughts* are specifically mentioned in this verse. God knows that it can be much easier to believe in our hearts that He is still there walking beside us, even though our minds can tell us otherwise.

Pull me through, Lord. My grasp is slipping! *~Lisa Copen*

Jesus Sees The Hurting

"As He went along, He saw a man blind from birth," (John 9:1).

Jesus passed by the man born blind, but He also "saw" him. It is so comforting to know that God sees us in our condition. For example, in Genesis, Chapter 16, after Sarah had dealt harshly with her maid Hagar, Hagar fled. Jesus found her after she had fled, however, and comforted her, giving direction to her in her affliction. She called God by the name, "Thou God seest me." She knew that God had seen her.

Jesus, on the day that His life would be changed forever, saw the man who was born blind. Beloved, God sees you in your affliction. You may feel all alone and that no one really understands or really cares about you in your chronic pain, but "nothing in all creation is hidden from God's sight," (Hebrews 4:13). God knows your physical needs. He sees you, and He longs to comfort you and care for you in the midst of your suffering.

Teresa of Avila, a saint in the 1500's, wrote, "Granting that we are always in the presence of God, yet it seems to me that those who pray are in His presence in a very different sense, for they, as it were, see that He is looking upon them, while others may be for days together without ever recollecting that God sees them."

No matter what you are going through, God sees you and all that concerns you. He wants to help. Not only does He want to comfort you in your affliction, but He also wants to bring meaning and purpose out of it. It is so much easier to endure chronic pain when we know that God is working His purpose and plan through the afflictions.

Jesus, I trust You are walking near me today and You see me in my affliction, just as You saw the blind man two thousand years ago. You want to help me in the midst of it. I surrender it over to You, Lord. Do with it as You wish. *~Virginia Ganskie*

Are You Dried Up?

". . .though in the morning it springs up new, by evening it is dry and withered," (Psalm 90:6).

Yesterday my husband and I got up at a decent time, but we were still wandering around at 11:30 a.m., trying to decide how to spend the day. "It is the fact that the sun hasn't come out yet," I remarked. "It feels like the day hasn't started."

I am blessed to live in San Diego, where the sun shines nearly every day. Moving from rainy Oregon to sunny Southern California, I quickly adjusted. I know that part of my ability to see the glory in every day is directly related to the fact that the sunshine gives me strength and hope. Our lives may have seemed to be filled with sunshine, and then illness arrived, causing daily challenges. Suddenly, it seems like we are waiting for life to start back up again. We are waiting for the sun to come back out.

Psalm 90:6, ". . .though in the morning it springs up new, by evening it is dry and withered," reminds me, however, that regardless of how bright or glorious the sunshine is, it quickly disappears. Here in San Diego, it has dried up everything, causing many families to lose their homes due to fire. Sunshine needs the rain. We need the storms to grow closer to our Lord. I recently picked up a large book filled with a collection of Andrew Murray's writings, the first one being *Abide in Christ.* "You did well to come," writes Murray. "You do better to abide. Who would, after seeking the King's palace, be content to stand in the door, when he is invited in to dwell in the King's presence and share with Him in all the glory of His royal life? Oh, let us enter and abide and enjoy to the full all the rich supply His wondrous love has prepared for us!"[40]

Lord, You bring sunshine into my life in so many ways, but I have become "dried up." Teach me to abide in You. You are my sunshine. You will protect me from feeling dried up. *~Lisa Copen*

My Hope Is In Jesus

"Brothers, we do not want you to be ignorant about those who fall asleep, or to grieve like the rest of men, who have no hope," (1 Thessalonians 4:13).

A friend shared with me the newest "cure" that she had discovered for her illness. I listened, smiled, and tried to appear encouraging. Yet, as she spoke, I remembered the many other times she had shared similar hopes with me, only to be devastated a few months later when the transformations were insignificant, if even existent.

There is nothing wrong with hoping for a cure. The vaccines and medications we have are a result of the drive that many people put forth to find a cure. Yet, when we put all of our hope into finding the cure, we tend to forget that God has already provided everything we need for our ultimate joy.

Simple words of Mother Goose say it clearly: "For every ailment under the sun, there is a remedy, or there is none; if there be one, try to find it; if there be none, never mind it." We can fall into the habit of worshiping cures and the quests for the cures instead of letting the researchers do their work, while we focus on Jesus. If there is none, never mind it!

Isaiah 48:10 says, "See, I have refined you, though not as silver; I have tested you in the furnace of affliction." Sometimes God puts us in the furnace. Rather than drawing closer to Him during the flames, we keep running for the fire hose or bucket of water to put out the fire. It's hard to "never mind it." It is a normal reaction, but God uses extraordinary circumstances.

1 Thessalonians 4:13 says, "Brothers, we do not want you to be ignorant about those who fall asleep, or to grieve like the rest of men, who have no hope." My ultimate hope is in You, Father. Putting my hope anywhere else would ultimately bring me grief.

~Lisa Copen

My Tent Is Going To Collapse

"Though an army besiege me, my heart will not fear; though war break out against me, even then will I be confident." (Psalms 27:3).

In my early twenties, I distinctly remember the day the Gulf War began. I left work and started the car. As Bette Midler's song *From a Distance*[41] came on the radio, I sat in the car and prayed for our soldiers, our nation, and for peace, as tears ran down my cheeks. Being a youngster during the Vietnam War, this was my first experience with our country truly at war.

Hearing the word "war" today no longer has the impact that it did then. I've not just grown accustomed to the new age in which we now reside, but I've also experienced a growing sense of God's power and control, over not just the nations, but the war within my own body.

There are days when I have a sense of fear when I think of living the rest of my life with a degenerative disease. Most of the time, however, I have a sense of peace about it all. Why? I have no logical answer other than God has blessed me with an understanding that He wants His best for me and He wants me to be willing to accept this. War is never pleasant. It is never easy. It seems every side pays a price. Thankfully, despite the fact that my body is at war against itself, attacking its own immune system, my Lord has already paid the price. Though I long for ease in doing the simple day-to-day things, it will never be. Yet I am without fear of the war that is going on in my body. I am confident! 1 Samuel 17:47 says, "For the battle is the Lord's...."

"For I am convinced that neither death nor life, neither angels nor demons, neither the present nor the future, nor any powers, neither height nor depth, nor anything else in all creation, will be able to separate [me] from the love of God that is in [You], Christ Jesus [my] Lord," (Romans 8:37-39). *~Lisa Copen*

Holding On To Victory

"For we wanted to come to you—certainly I, Paul, did, again and again—but Satan stopped us," (1 Thessalonians 2:18).

I desperately wanted to go to a writer's conference; after months of being on a waiting list, I was accepted. Then I began to flare, making the drive nearly impossible and the goals of the week crumble. I realized that God was saying "no." Or... was it Satan attacking? When Satan is unable to destroy the dream, he tries to destroy the dreamer.

When we live with physical limitations, there are often times when we want to do something, and yet we are unable to do it. Circumstances are thrown up against us, preventing us from fulfilling commitments and, at times, our dreams. Last week, on my way to a meeting at the church, it poured rain, and my fingers felt like sausages as my whole body flared. I dreaded a long day in one chair. It took everything in me not to turn my car around, go back home and crawl into bed. And then I realized how incredible the meeting must be if Satan was trying to weaken my earlier enthusiasm.

As my life intertwines with ministry, I see the depth of the challenges. They are overwhelming, and I feel a direct spiritual attack. People assure me, "It's a compliment that Satan is attacking!" Logically I realize that, but in my heart I feel, *Lord, if this is Your will, why are You allowing it to be so difficult? If You can turn water into wine, You can fix this!*

Do you feel the attack and recognize it for what it is? Even the dedicated Apostle Paul had plans disrupted. He recognized Satan's attack on the ministry. It's heartwarming to focus on Christ and avoid "the other side," but we must recognize our enemy. He will *not* get the victory.

Lord, my plans may not go the way that I wish, but I will cling to You and enjoy the freedom of knowing that my heart, soul, and mind are in Your hands. You will have the last word. ~Lisa Copen

He Knows Our Limits

"He knows our frame; He remembers we are dust," (Psalm 103:14).

Those of us struggling with chronic pain and illness often feel we are carrying a burden that can quickly become overwhelming. We are often in pain; many times we cannot complete tasks we would like to accomplish. We deal with doctors, medications, insurance, folks who don't understand, and the many financial concerns related to long-term illness. We may begin to wonder if God knows how much we can bear.

I read a story that made me think differently. A father wanted to move a steel beam that weighed three hundred pounds, so he asked his son to grab the other end and help him set it in place. The young man tried to lift his end of the huge beam, but he could not. In fact, he ended up in the hospital. The father was heartbroken and realized, because of his own strength, he had overlooked his son's weakness. However, we must remember that our Heavenly Father will never overlook His children's weaknesses, for "He knows our frame; He remembers that we are dust," (Psalm 103:13).

Whenever you feel you are under a heavy load or burden, take comfort in the knowledge that the Lord God will never give you more to carry than you can endure. God knows our load limit, and He graciously limits our load. Just trust Him to be faithful. "The problem of pain will have no ultimate solution until God recreates the earth," writes Philip Yancey. "I am sustained by faith in that great hope."[42] "The Lord is gracious and righteous; our God is full of compassion," (Psalm 116:5).

Heavenly Father, when I feel overwhelmed with trials, help me to remember that You will never burden me with more than I can carry with Your help. All I need to do is ask You to be with me in all my trials, and You will help me carry my load.

~Patricia Armstrong

Becoming Childlike

"...unless you change and become like little children, you will never enter the kingdom of heaven'" (Matthew 18:3).

I recently heard this story about my little cousin: "My husband and I had been teaching our three-year-old son to use a tissue when he sneezed. Too often, he would reach for his sleeve. Each time he sneezed, we would say, 'God bless you.' Then we'd encourage him to get a tissue or frantically try to get one to him before he wiped his nose on his shirt. Last week, Zachary had a cold and was sneezing often. There was a lot of blessing going on in our home. Sitting there one evening, he sneezed hard. He looked down at his arm and said, 'Mommy, I've got God-bless-you all over my sleeve.'"

Does living with chronic illness zap away your innocence? We've become more educated than we wish on hospital check-in procedures or how to interpret lab results and. We have our prescription refill numbers memorized. We hear more about our nurses' families than our own. God desires us to have the innocence of a child, the belief that, as our parent, He will take care of everything. He wants us to be able to fall asleep at night with the joy that we had when a parent tucked us in. For some of us, God is the only parent we have had who has tucked us in and offered comfort. Life is overwhelming. Faith can become complicated. Joy becomes a mystery. For today, try to have the innocence of a child. Laugh at the simple things in life. Believe that everything is going to be okay.

God, You know I love a good mystery, or why would You have chosen to tell me about heaven in these words? "Listen, I tell you a mystery: We will not all sleep, but we will all be changed—in a flash, in the twinkling of an eye, at the last trumpet. For the trumpet will sound, the dead will be raised imperishable, and we will be changed," (1 Corinthians 15:51,52). You truly do have the whole world in Your hands. Regardless of the gunk in my life, You are still blessing me.

~Lisa Copen

For Such A Time As This

"And who knows but that you have come to royal position for such a time as this?" (Esther 4:14b).

In the building where I live, over a hundred people reside in hospital beds or wheelchairs. They have suffered from strokes, paralysis, and some will be here for years. In the ten years I have lived here, I've seen many roommates leave on gurneys—on their way to the mortuary.

I'm sure when Esther was growing up, she never imagined that she would become a queen. As queen, perhaps she looked at her royal robes and shook her head in amazement that such a thing could happen to her. A plot to sentence Jews to death was discovered by Esther's uncle. He begged her to plead with the king to save the Jews. "Who knows but that you have come to royal position for such a time as this?" I can relate to Esther. Growing up, I never imagined I would end up on a ventilator and live in a care center. I often shake my head in amazement that such a thing could happen to me. I wonder, have I come to this center for such a time as this?

Here I sit, wholly desiring to be elsewhere, but God has allowed me to be here. Could it be for such a time as this? While people around me sit in despair, I know hope from experiencing the true Comforter. While they search for answers, I live my life for the Author of Truth. Has God allowed me to be here to shine His light in the darkness? I marvel when I think of the people God has allowed me to minister to. One woman came here with burns covering ninety percent of her body; the fire claimed the lives of two of her children. Through friendship and Bible studies, I was able to point her to the hope and comfort found in God alone.

Father, may I be like Esther and continue to use my circumstances to bring deliverance! You have allowed me to be where I am now. How can I serve You from where I am? ~*Jason R. Mitchener*

The Shallow End Of The Pool

"...We consider blessed those who have persevered. You have heard of Job's perseverance and have seen what the Lord finally brought about. The Lord is full of compassion and mercy," (James 5:11).

Swimming lessons generally weren't bad. I was the kind of child, however, that put up with the teachers throwing rings into the pool and telling me to retrieve them simply because my mom promised a stop at Dairy Queen for a cherry Dilly Bar ® afterwards. At the end of every swimming season, we were forced to jump off the diving board at the deep end of the pool. I left the fun floating toys at the shallow end and had to go to the board, where someone would push me off if I refused to jump... which happened more than once.

Helen Keller once said, "Character cannot be developed in ease and quiet. Only through experience of trial and suffering can the soul be strengthened, vision cleared, ambition inspired, and success achieved." I've experienced firsthand the joy that can come from pain. As loved ones around me go through difficulties with coworkers, illnesses, and more, I can empathize, but more importantly, I can reassure them that there is light at the end. What a joy it is to receive that phone call six months later and hear a voice of someone I love who has experienced the furnace and is now reaping the rewards of being a new person in Christ.

I still don't like the fires. I didn't like the deep end of the pool. I don't enjoy being pruned, trimmed, molded, or scolded. There are simply better ways I can think of to spend my days, but then I wouldn't be receiving God's best for my life. I wouldn't be in His will. I wouldn't reap the benefits that outweigh the cost.

"Test me in this," [You say, O Lord,] "and see if I will not throw open the floodgates of heaven and pour out so much blessing that you will not have room enough for it," (Malachi 3:10b). Okay, Lord, I'll jump!

~Lisa Copen

Surrendering The Mind Too

"...offer your bodies as living sacrifices, holy and pleasing to God—this is your spiritual act of worship. Do not conform any longer to the pattern of this world, but be transformed by the renewing of your mind. Then you will be able to test and approve what God's will is—His good, pleasing and perfect will." (Romans 12:1-2).

How I have longed for the renewing of my mind. A stroke eight months ago has left my mind in a jumble. It's filled with muddle, confusion, and a disorganized mess of thoughts.

As I read Romans 12, I find hope and direction. It's exciting to realize that my body, regardless of its condition, is holy and pleasing to God. When I offer myself to Him as a living sacrifice, in a spiritual act of worship, no longer conforming to any worldly patterns, I am transformed! My mind is renewed. His will is made known to me. I can be of service to Him just the way I am. What a marvelous revelation!

Most of us take great pride in our ability to speak with eloquence and to sound educated and informed. It's a humbling experience to find one's self grasping for the right word or recalling a small fact. While once I could speak articulately with ease and have words freely flow off of my tongue, these simple things do not happen as naturally now. How I long to praise the Holy God with confidence in my abilities. God will work through my weaknesses, however, not my strengths. I must humbly allow it. By faith, I am putting it into writing: In coming months I plan to use my gift as a writer in proportion to my faith and according to God's grace given to me.

Today I reclaim the gift that You have given me. "We have different gifts, according to the grace given us," (Romans 12:6). Lord, don't allow my pride about my abilities to get in the way of doing the ministry that You would have me to do. *~Nancy Wilcox*

God Remembers You

"But God remembered Noah," (Genesis 8:1).

God remembered Noah. Oh, how I love those words! Noah, his family, and two of every species of animals, had been protected in the ark while the flood destroyed everything on the earth. The storm raged, and after it was all over, "God remembered Noah."

Dear one, God remembers you! Sometimes this may be hard to believe as our struggles go on endlessly, without apparent improvement. Indeed, some of us may be actually getting worse, and we silently wonder, *God, are You really there? Can I really believe that You still care about me since You are not easing my pain or giving me the strength to do all of the things that really need to be done – even for You?*

If God ever sets us free from pain or illness, it will be in His perfect timing. He won't allow a healing to happen a moment too soon for what He intends to accomplish through our suffering. I know... it's hard to hear this.

Although you may think that you cannot endure much more, remember that God has not forgotten you! Let us listen to His Word: "But Zion said, 'The Lord has forsaken me, the Lord has forgotten me.' [And the Lord said]: Can a mother forget the baby at her breast and have no compassion on the child she has borne? Though she may forget, I will not forget you!" (Isaiah 49:14-15).

Jesus died on the cross for you. You were engraved on the palms of His hands, and He lives for you each day. No, Beloved, a thousand times, no; He has not forgotten you.

Lord, the pain that I have had to endure will someday be turned into a blessing that I never could have dreamed possible, and I will tell others, "See, the Lord did not forget me, and He won't forget you either." Help me be patient in the process. *~Virginia Ganskie*

The Heart Where Deep Waters Tread

"The purposes of a man's heart are deep waters, but a man of understanding draws them out," (Proverbs 20:5).

My husband is a thinker, and I am a talker. I speak before I think and am content if I have an audience for my story. I recently read the following advice: "If you are telling a story and someone interrupts you, don't continue with the story. If people really want to hear it, they will ask you to continue." I ask you, what fun is this? Most of us have a friend or loved one whom we must draw out if they are to really talk to us. It is so easy to get caught up in our own life—dealing with challenges, disappointments, and the daily pain—that it can become easy to forget that it takes time to sit and just listen.

As newlyweds, when my husband would walk through the door, I would ask, "How was your day?" He disliked this question, and he would answer "fine." I'd say, "Fine? What was wrong?" "Nothing! I said it was fine," he'd reply. For him, fine is a nine on a scale of one to ten; but for me, it's a two. However, I have learned to just wait patiently for him to share about his day.

Job's friends did something right; they sat for seven days before saying a word. Seven days! If you read the book of Job, you will discover that Job wished they had continued to sit quietly and refrain from offering advice. I find sitting quietly beside a hurting friend a challenge. As much as I personally grow weary of people approaching me with cures and potions, I still want to fix the lives of those around me who are hurting. To draw someone's feelings out, however, to let them know that we genuinely care about what is going on in their lives, we must take the time to sit, listen, and speak gently, hearing their needs, not fulfilling our desires to fix it.

Father, help me listen and not try to carry the conversation. Help me to be quiet so I can hear Your voice. *~Lisa Copen*

Onward Christian Soldiers

"Consider it pure joy, my brothers, whenever you face trials of many kinds, because you know that the testing of your faith develops perseverance," (James 1:2-3).

"Hang in there! Keep on keeping on! Go for the gold! Keep your eyes on the goal!" All are encouragements to endure our present struggles. Living with chronic pain, we especially need this encouragement to keep going. Day after day, our struggles seem to be without end. The joy James is speaking of in the verse above has to be supernatural, coming only through the strength and power of the Holy Spirit living in us.

Does that mean we smile at every turn in our lives? Does that mean we laugh with every pain or every difficulty we encounter in our disabled lives? No, I don't think so. It means having a peaceful heart, trusting in the Lord God, knowing that He knows what it means to suffer because He died for our sins at Calvary. Jesus persevered through such agony for us, to the point of sweating drops of blood, so that we would inherit eternal life with Him.

What gracious and precious love! It is more than we can comprehend. "I pray God may open your eyes and let you see what hidden treasures He bestows on us in the trials from which the world thinks only to flee," says John of the Cross.[43] "He predestined us to be adopted as His sons through Jesus Christ, in accordance with His pleasure and will," (Ephesians 1:5).

O God, Your love and Your good pleasure—that is why I can persevere through my trials with joy. Since You have loved me, I have the same power that Jesus had. Onward Christian soldiers!

~Holly Baker

I Feel So Slow

"So let my Lord go on ahead of His servant, while I move along slowly at the pace of the droves before me. . . " (Genesis 33:14).

I'm not one who lollygags, but wherever I go, I feel like I am moving in slow motion. Today, a car stopped, and the driver let me walk across the street while he waited. I felt as though he was staring at me, wondering why I was moving so slowly when he had been kind enough to wait for me to cross. I don't appear to have a physical ailment; people tend to assume that I am tired or lazy. *I'm actually running!* I want to yell to those waiting. *I'm not dillydallying!*

In Genesis 33, I find that Jacob understood that at times a slower pace is for the best. Esau wanted to get his herd to Seir quickly, but Jacob knew that, if he pushed the animals beyond their capabilities, he would risk losing them in death. The animals needed to be allowed to move at a slower pace than the rest of the crowd, and then they would arrive safely. I believe most everyone who lives with illness copes with the feelings of inadequacy of accomplishment.

Andrew Murray wrote, "Have you ever noticed the difference in the Christian life between work and fruit? A machine can do work; only life can bear fruit."[44] How true it is that we are God's living children who can bear fruit in our lives regardless of what "work" we do for Him and regardless of our abilities, or even our disabilities.

Pace counts, and in Your eyes, Lord, slower is usually the better pace. "It is good to wait quietly for the salvation of the Lord," (Lamentations 3:26). It may take me longer to get somewhere than it once did, but I can still get there. It can be tempting to compare myself with those around me who have a much faster pace, but speed doesn't matter. I will get there, and then, like Jacob, I will offer thanks to You that I made it at all. *~Lisa Copen*

It's Not the Season For Figs

"Seeing in the distance a fig tree in leaf, he went to find out if it had any fruit. When he reached it, he found nothing but leaves, because it was not the season for figs," (Mark 11:13).

When I was diagnosed with illness, I challenged God: *So what are You going to do with this? Go ahead, show me!* Well, He showed me in a way I could not have ever imagined by calling my heart to the ministry of chronic illness. Okay, so I was a good sport about the illness thing, so surely God would give me the other desires of my heart; right? Wrong.

Years after beginning the path to have a child, my husband and I still aimlessly walk the toy aisles, talking about "maybe someday." Regardless of the blessings God has bestowed upon us, we still have a desire for that which we do not have. It is too easy to count our misfortunes as we see others' successes; to look at our bodies with resentment as we see others run without effort or live without appreciation.

I tend to fill vacations with reading materials that focus on marketing your business or growing in the Lord. I feel, if I give myself a few moments to let my mind wander, it will take me to a place where my circumstances will just hurt too much. Reading and planning enables my thoughts to wander to God's future plans, rather than focus on my current situation. We will often wander to whatever fig tree we think will hold our dreams and fulfill our desires… but we find it bare. It is not full of answered dreams, pain-free moments, or miracles. It is without figs; but remember, it's still a fig tree. It is simply not the season for figs. God has not chopped down the tree; our empty-handed moments are only a season.

Lord, teach me to remember that, despite what I may not have this season, I do have You, and You are the only thing that I need. Remind me that my tree still has leaves. You are watering it. Another season will be here soon, and You will have my fig tree bloom and produce fruit. *~Lisa Copen*

I'm Tired Of Being Patient

"What strength do I have, that I should still hope? What prospects, that I should be patient?" (Job 6:11).

My doctor has run out of treatments to try for one of my conditions. Today, the nurse called and said, "The doctor would like you to see someone else. She doesn't know what else to do." I feel helpless, even hopeless. It is so frustrating when you feel that those whom you have trusted are passing you off to someone else, forcing you to start the cycle again. I call a new doctor to make an appointment, and of course, the first thing the receptionist asks is, "Are you a new patient?" dooming me into an extended wait despite my insistence that it is an urgent matter. It's times like this I cry out to God, "What strength do I have, that I should still hope? What prospects, that I should be patient?"

Chronic illness is not pleasant. Pain is not something I would have chosen. However, I have grown accustomed to it. It is the never-ending list of side effects and new symptoms, such as the ones I am experiencing now, that get me down. When a morning ritual consists of lotions and pills, vitamins and more pills, I grow weary. When walking becomes nearly impossible and rising from a chair becomes a workout, my spirit wilts. *Where are You, Lord? What lesson am I not learning?*

"The point is clear," writes Robert Schuller. "Nobody is free from problems. A problem-free life is an illusion—a mirage in the desert. It is a dangerously deceptive perception, which can mislead, blind, and distract. Every problem holds positive possibilities. 'It is the glory of God to conceal a thing,' (Proverbs 25:20). Every problem contains secret ingredients of some creative potential either for yourself of someone else."[45]

You who shaped the heavens are shaping my life, so I can reply, "I know that You can do all things; no plan of Yours can be thwarted," (Job 42:2).

~Lisa Copen

Guide Your Sails To Jesus

"Though I walk in the midst of trouble, You preserve my life; You stretch out Your hand against the anger of my foes, with Your right hand You save me," (Psalm 138:7).

Corrie ten Boom once said, "Is prayer your steering wheel or your spare tire?"[46] I have a picture in my bedroom that states the following: "Lord, guide my steps in ways of grace that they may ever be in harmony to the music which you have set this world."

When I look at this picture and say this prayer, I know that my day is off to the right start. God is always there, listening twenty-four hours a day, seven days a week. He understands the pain and frustrations we feel. God became man incarnate in the person of Jesus; Christ was fully human and fully divine. He knows the agony and pains we feel, and therefore, we have a Savior we can identify with.

Tim Hansel, author of *You Gotta Keep Dancin'*, says there are two reasons people miss joy: one, they have preconceived images of what joy is supposed to be, and two, they try to cling to those experiences, to keep and preserve them.

"So do not fear, for I am with you; do not be dismayed, for I am your God. I will strengthen you, and I will help you. I will uphold you with My righteous right hand," (Isaiah 41:10).

When the storms of life surround you,
and your soul is like a restless sea,
Guide your sails to Jesus,
To the God of Calvary. *(K. DeCarlo)*

Jesus, You know how to calm my heart and let me experience joy! I trust You will restore my soul and lead me to a new understanding of who You are. Lord Jesus, guide my paths this day and fill my heart with Your divine love and peace that will never pass away.

~Kay DeCarlo

Healing The Hurts That Hold Us

"Bear with each other and forgive whatever grievances you may have against one another. Forgive as the Lord forgave you," (Colossians 3:13).

At a recent fibromyalgia conference, I spoke with a young woman who sat near me at lunch. Although her mother tried to offer her comfort, she shared, her mom had some skepticism about the illness' existence. "My father told me that he didn't want to have contact with me until I stopped being a hypochondriac." She looked so defeated.

"Though my father and mother forsake me, the Lord will receive me," (Psalm 27:10). Living with chronic illness is difficult. Living with the assumptions, opinions, and hurts that others communicate with us, however, hurts even more than the pain. And yet, are we called to forgive? To act like everything is okay? We are called to forgive so our own hearts can be at peace. We are not called to be doormats or put ourselves in harm's way. God wants us to grow closer to Him; if we are holding in hurts, He will not be able to come near to us to fully heal our heart and its wounds.

H. Norman Wright once wrote, "Forgiveness is no longer allowing what has happened to poison you."[47] I agree. Forgiveness is not condoning that a person's acts were appropriate or acceptable. Forgiveness is not being the weaker party and allowing the person to hurt you again. Forgiveness is letting go of the need to hold a grudge and allowing God to do what He wants with your hurts.

Has someone said something that hurt? Has someone reached out with criticism, not comfort? Has a phone call ended with tears? Did the phone call that you hoped for never come? There is one who will always comfort.

God, come into my heart and repair the damage. Only You can make the hurts truly be healed. ~*Lisa Copen*

X-Ray Vision

"O Lord, You have searched me and You know me. You know when I sit and when I rise; You perceive my thoughts from afar. You discern my going out and my lying down; You are familiar with all my ways," (Psalm 139:1-3).

My doctor placed the x-ray before me and pointed to my shoulder, where the ball fits into the socket, explaining why I needed a shoulder replacement. No cartilage remained, and bone was rubbing against bone, causing pain and continuing damage. I was amazed at what a simple x-ray could reveal about the human body. Externally, there was no visible sign of what was happening internally. Silently, I asked God to lead me to the right decision regarding surgery.

In Psalm 139, David becomes aware of God's all-encompassing "x-ray vision." He is amazed at God's level of comprehension. He realizes that God knew everything about him before he was even born. No matter what David does and no matter where he goes, the Lord sees all and knows all. God is concerned with David's physical being; but more so, his heart and soul. David acknowledges God's omniscience and asks the Father to lead him in the way everlasting. God's hedge of protection surrounds David, and His hand is always upon him. Through serious mistakes in David's life, God still sees what others cannot; David is a man after God's heart.

In the days that followed my visit to the doctor, God exposed and calmed my fears. He helped me decide in favor of surgery. He showed me that His protective hedge is not limited to David, but is there for all who seek Him.

Father, Your protective hedge surrounds me, and I am at peace. Thank You for leading me in Your way, according to Your plan.

~Nancy Wilcox

Walking The Walk– In A Wheelchair

"The good man brings good things out of the good stored up in his heart, and the evil man brings evil things out of the evil stored up in his heart. For out of the overflow of his heart his mouth speaks," (Luke 6:45).

Having lived in many areas of the United States, it is the South that frustrates me the most. I'm called "Honey" and "Sugar" in the grocery checkout line, but once I am in the parking lot, my wheelchair is in the way. People openly stare at those with disabilities yet claim to be warm and friendly.

I must, however, consider myself to also be incongruent. I can write devotions and talk about feeling well adjusted; yet when someone stares at me, my fist balls up in anger. I consider myself a Christian and preach to others without realizing I need to do some work on myself. When a lady runs up to me in the store and rudely questions what is wrong, or the person at the gym steps in front of me and demands to know why I use a wheelchair, my gut instinct, or my sin instinct, is to tell them what I really think.

The anger rolls off my brain, and I want so badly to revert to my old ways, but illness and pain are not an excuse to be hurtful to others. We can tell the truth in love, as the Bible says, but it is not open season on inflicting pain. Justice is not mine; vengeance does not belong to me.

The Bible says that what comes from my mouth really comes from my heart. It is a window into what is stored there. Before I reveal my true sin nature to someone by being rude, it's better to stop and say a prayer.

Lord, I don't want to allow others to win the battle by hurting me with their comments, stares, or inappropriate questions. Help me rise above it, and let them see the Love of Christ instead. Help me speak the truth but speak it with love. *~Rebecca Koszalinski*

Showing Up

"When evening came, Jesus arrived..." (Mark 14:17).

I attended the same small church from the time I could walk until I left for college. To this day, the pastor, simply known as Norm, shakes your hand as you leave, and on a cold Christmas Eve, one will find a Tootsie Roll® treat swept from a hidden pocket in his black robe into your hand. For years, he drove a purple '55 Ford pickup. If you were to peek under his robe on a Sunday morning, chances are you would find jeans and a purple sweatshirt. I've attended many large churches that have "worship teams," "staff counselors," and "baptisms at La Jolla." I have seen few hearts like Norm's.

Large churches sometimes find it inconvenient to establish programs for the homebound; they worry over insurance regulations and have to get elders' approval to go into homes. Norm simply went. For years, after he was done reading the morning paper, he would take it over to an elderly lady's home, and she would have hot raisin bread waiting. It wasn't about the paper; it was about the fellowship. Much of Norm's ministry is about showing up.

Norm didn't visit others because he had nothing else to do. He served on the school board for years, raised two sons and two daughters, and was at every football game and basketball game I cheered for. When I was in high school, he led the high school Sunday school class before church. He bought Girl Scout cookies from me as a child and raffle tickets when I was a cheerleader. He bent over to hold the hands of those that could no longer stand for worship. He still grasps the attention of young ones by mentioning a Sunday cartoon in his sermon. He humbly serves, always with joy and laughter. His authenticity and vulnerability to allow God to use him is what we need in more churches today. Too few just show up.

Help me show up to serve You, even when it hurts. *~Lisa Copen*

Finding Streams In The Desert

"I am making a way in the desert and streams in the wasteland." (Isaiah 43:19).

One of my favorite classical devotionals is L.B. Cowman's *Streams in the Desert,* and I have plumbed the depths of this rich book repeated times in the last two decades, but never with more fervor and focus than since my multiple sclerosis diagnosis. One writer gripped me as he described the "wounds of nature." He spoke of them as the broken things, crushed things, and the burnt things—the wheat that is crushed to make bread; the incense that is burnt in order to release its pungent fragrance. Even the earth is broken by unrelenting blows of the plow, enabling seed to enter. All of nature knows that brokenness—death itself—is necessary for new life to spring forth.

We hesitate to imitate what we see in all of creation, not certain we can bear the pain brokenness leaves as its "calling card." Chronic illness crushes us, burns us, and breaks us. Instead of embracing its blows, we argue and analyze. We doubt and deny. Where is redemption for my un-doneness? And the earth, seed, and incense smile. They only know God's goodness; we question it. They are content with God's ways; we contend them. They experience resurrection life: bread from brokenness, fragrance from fire, produce from plowing. Oh, that we would recognize what creation has reveled in throughout eternity past and present: God is good, and what He does is good, (Psalm 119:68).

Lord, as I grieve and grapple, wait and wonder, always remind me that You are masterful and You will always provide a stream in my wasteland. You take my waste, brokenness, and weakness and redeem them with Your resurrectional power, at work in those who believe. I can trust You. All of nature does. Hallelujah! What a Savior!

~Connie Kennemer

What Will The Tests Show?

"He will have no fear of bad news; his heart is steadfast, trusting in the Lord," (Psalms 112:7).

The weekend is long when you are waiting for test results. The two days seem to go by so slowly, as if each tick of the clock desires to distress me. I should trust the Lord that everything is going to be okay. He understands that I can't handle anymore; right? The pain has changed my entire life, and now I am faced with another hurdle I must jump. I am tired of fighting. I am numb with fear. I am so scared about what is in my future.

Where are You, Lord? I want to cry out. *Why are You allowing this evil to attack my body one more time? Have I not given You enough already? Do I not surrender my life to You every day?*

I'm usually more positive. Once, I knew people who had conquered illnesses, but now, I know more people who have not been able to overcome them despite their attempts. I have witnessed how unfair life can be, and this frightens me.

Sister Mary Tricky once said, "Fear is faith that it won't work out." As I wait, I must pray for God to restore my strength for whatever I discover tomorrow. I will ask that He take away my fear. I will not fear God's plan for my life. Each of us faces an unknown future. Despite our goals, plans, and even our actions, it is always God who is in control, not us.

Alexander MacLaren wrote, "Each of us may be sure that if God sends us on stony paths, He will provide us with strong shoes, and He will not send us out on any journey for which He does not equip us well."

Lord, remind me that my prayer to hear good test results tomorrow is no bigger of a request than for a close parking spot. You are the Almighty, and so I have nothing to fear. *~Lisa Copen*

The Purification

"Remove the dross from the silver, and out comes material for the silversmith," (Proverbs 25:4).

Webster's Dictionary defines "dross" as "scum that forms on the surface of molten metal," "waste or foreign matter," or "impurities."[48] God made us in His image, pure and perfect, but sin has left us riddled with impurities. It is God's desire that we "be holy as He is holy," (Leviticus 11:44). And one of the ways the Lord purifies us is through suffering. "Consider it pure joy... whenever you face trials of many kinds," (James 1:2). It's hard to understand why we should be happy when difficulties come our way, but James explains that trouble, when faced with Jesus at our side, will help us to become "mature and complete."

For myself, living with chronic health problems has burned off the dross of self-reliance. I used to live independently of the Lord, relying on my own limited abilities and questionable wisdom instead of seeking His will in all things. Suffering has also burned off my pride. Since illness has taken from me the ability to work for a living and to pursue a number of activities, I can no longer point to my accomplishments and say, "Look what I have done!" Now, getting through a day successfully means leaning on Jesus. Now, I point to "my" accomplishments and say, "Look what the Lord has done!"

I also had the flaw of self-centeredness. I was never a mean person, but I certainly didn't have the understanding and compassion which poor health has given me. That was one more bit of dross that had to go to make me material that God could use. He really couldn't work with someone who lived apart from Him and who was puffed up with pride and who didn't bear His love for others in her heart.

Lord, You have used suffering to change me. It hasn't been easy, but it certainly has been worthwhile! *~Mary Lou Cornish*

Is There Any Hope?

"He tears me down on every side till I am gone; He uproots my hope like a tree," (Job 19:10).

As I sign in at the doctor's office, the receptionist asks the doctor if he is ready for me. He replies, "It's Miss Fatty Cheeks." Despite my dismay, I say, "That really hurt. I am not going to come back here if you continue to say things like that." He apologizes and says, "I was just teasing."

"I like you," I continue. "You can tell me how you feel, and I can tell you how I feel, but there is a line, and you just crossed it." He's surprised and embarrassed; his office staff has just heard him be reprimanded by me, a patient. It had to be said. He knows that I am a Christian and that I am easygoing and forgiving. He has now learned that I am not a doormat for his moods. His comment hurt. And all I can think of are the many spirits he has crushed by his inconsiderate teasing.

After a year of Prednisone, I began to have the the visible side effects that I dreaded: the puffy face and the weight gain. Months earlier, my doctor told me not to worry about the cosmetic effects of the drugs, but to think about what my body needed. I relented, regretting the choice. On this day, however, he uprooted my hope. I wanted to cry, but with God's strength, I chose to tell him how I felt.

People will come into our lives who will try to uproot our hope. We may even feel like God is the one uprooting our hope since He's allowed these discouraging comments. But our Father is the only one we can turn to in the midst of these moments. He will be our tree of life, keeping us rooted to Him at all times. C. Neil Strait once said, "A man can go on without wealth, and even without purpose, for a while. But he will not go on without hope."

What a wonderful gift Your presence is. My hope shall not be uprooted by anyone when You're my foundation. ~*Lisa Copen*

Winter's Storm

"My comfort in my suffering is this: Your promise preserves my life," (Psalm 119:50).

My soul is aching from without. . ..within,
Tossed about like a leaf in the wind.
Searching for grounding, it twists and turns,
Restless and brittle. . .
For rest it yearns. . . .

Storms through the days and nights soak me through;
My tears flow as I search,
Desperately for You.
Gently You speak to my heart and dry my tears,
Taking my hand as I work through my fears.

Your angels surround me,
and bear up my soul.
As day after day,
I'm in turmoil and toil.

My blinded eyes are opening,
As His ways become more clear.
My broken heart is mending,
As His love becomes more dear.

"My child," I finally hear Him say,
"I've waited for you to come,
with trust and faith in hand.
So I could strengthen that measure ten-fold,
As you travel this troubled land."

"So much more you need to grow,
and to become more like Me,"
He said with a loving smile.
"This trial is but only for a little while.
Oh! How I trust that you will see!"

"For My heart aches for you, My child,
As I see your tears and heartache flow.
But a stronger person you will emerge
As you learn to just let go!"

So now my faith is growing stronger,
As I try so hard to thank Him
for this painful season.
But grow through this, I must
to emerge a stronger person for this reason.

Someday I will look back on these growing days,
and I'll praise Him for the love He's shown.
As He's taught me to trust His purpose,
and willingly acknowledge His ways.

The sun will soon shine once again,
As its brightened warmth sends healing within.
My soul shall smile as I lift my praise,
Towards Heaven's open ceiling!

~Ellie. M. O'Steen

A Quiet Life

"Make it your ambition to lead a quiet life. . . ." (1 Thessalonians 4:11a).

I woke up today feeling a bit lonely. My house is quiet, and the rain is coming down, making it dark and dreary. It is one of those days when I wish I had a friend who would just drop by. I could serve a cup of tea in my new teacups, and we could reminisce about warmer days and discuss the forthcoming spring. Instead, I face a day of laundry that needs washing, dishes that need scrubbing and floors that need mopping. If I had the energy to do all of those household duties, I wouldn't mind, but knowing that the exhaustion will set in soon after I shower drains my spirit.

Oh, Lord. Do You understand how I feel? I ask. Only moments later, as I am reading my Bible, I come to the verse, "Make it your ambition to lead a quiet life. . . ." *My ambition, Lord? But I am not a quiet kind of person. I want to have a loud life, full of excitement and adventure!* "Make it your ambition to lead a quiet life," I read again. On days such as today, when I want to be able to focus on my accomplishments and get together with friends, God has called me to live a quiet life. For today, I will focus on this verse in which God spoke to me. I will reflect on what it means to live a quiet life.

It's not a life I would have chosen, but God knows that it's a life in which I will grow closer to Him; that is what He values. "Let's never forget," says Elisabeth Elliot, "that some of God's greatest mercies are His refusals. He says no in order that He may, in some way we cannot imagine, say yes. All His ways with us are merciful. His meaning is always love."[49] When we are swept up in cooking, cleaning, entertaining, carpooling, appointments, returning calls, and nurturing those around us, it's difficult to remember quiet living.

For today, God, You have given me the gift of living a quiet life and remembering that is it to be my ambition. ~*Lisa Copen*

Persistence And Leaning On God

"In all your ways acknowledge Him, and He will direct your paths," (Proverbs 3:6).

I recently had the pleasure of spending a quiet week on the beaches of Cape Cod, in a quaint cottage. While lying on the beach, listening to the ebb and flow of the waves, the tide pounded gently upon the ocean's shore. I spotted a family of five sandpipers flying just above the salt of the wave's tide.

The sandpipers circled and then landed on the beach. They began looking for food. As soon as they would place their beaks in the sand for food, a wave would come and wash their tracks away. When the waves would come, the sandpipers would scurry along, almost communicating, "Oh no, there goes our chance!"

Once again, however, they would persistently try to seek for food, pecking their beaks into the sand, only to scurry along once the waves came in around them covering their tracks again. "Persistent little birds," I thought. "A lot like us." We, like sandpipers, often look for things in the same manner. Waves come upon us when faced with adversity, pain, or sickness, yet we persevere. How? By the grace of God.

I find myself becoming more like that persistent sandpiper. Lately, however, I hear God telling me He wants me to be more like a lamb—an obedient, humble lamb of His Fold, who listens to His call and does what He says. *Do not worry about tomorrow. When worry sets in, toss it aside and pray. Give it all to me, the Shepherd of your Heart.* And so, that is my prayer, that Jesus will be always the Shepherd of my heart and yours, and that He will lead you in the paths that you should go.

Lord, don't let the crashing waves of life discourage me for a moment!

~Kay DeCarlo

Life Is Short

"Show me, O Lord, my life's end and the number of my days; let me know how fleeting is my life. You have made my days a mere handbreadth; the span of my years is as nothing before You. Each man's life is but a breath," (Psalm 39:4,5).

I have a friendship I delight in. A mutual friend suggested that Connie and I meet. Soon, I received a note from Connie, explaining that she had multiple sclerosis and was a Christian. I smiled to myself when I read that; we already had two driving forces in our life in common: God and illness. It was her invitation to a coffee house, however, that really caught my attention. Unlike most of the people I knew with chronic illness, *she drank coffee!*

When I met Connie, she laughed at my comments and said, "Life is short. I like coffee." I'd found a kindred spirit, and nearly ten years later, she has become my mentor, encourager, listener, advisor, and when needed, rear-kicker. Laughs and lattes, mixed in with many tears and prayers, have given me something precious to cling to in the dark moments of living with illness.

Not a day passes when I am not reminded of how short life is. It seems the pain will never go away, but in reality, the pain will one day disappear. Life is short. Our world goes on. Bodies will quit. Wars will start. Hurricanes will rip apart homes. Divorces will shatter families… but life is so short. Every day I must remind myself of this fact when I become too focused on the insignificant details. I have much to be thankful for. I have many people I must tell, "I love you" and, "Thank you." There are so many things I have to do, I don't know where to begin. I don't even have time to consider my physical limitations. I need to make a list. . . how much better I could concentrate with a nice cup of coffee.

"Show me, O Lord, my life's end and the number of my days; let me know how fleeting is my life," (Psalm 39:4). *~Lisa Copen*

Building Faith, Page By Page

"Consequently, faith comes from hearing the message, and the message is heard through the Word of Christ," (Romans 10:1).

At times, I've been tempted to doubt God. When I was first hooked up to a ventilator, I doubted that God loved me. How could a loving God let me suffer so much? My faith shrank to nothingness, and I turned my back on the Lord.

When I got sick, I stopped reading my Bible. I didn't have the physical strength to turn the pages anymore. Now, as I look back, I see a connection that I missed then: the less I read the Bible, the more my faith shrank.

I really had no excuse for not getting into God's Word. I could have listened to the Bible on tape or had a friend read the Bible to me. But I didn't do any of these things, and my faith shriveled. Reading God's Word builds our faith. We see how God worked before and acknowledge He still works the same way today. God does not change.

When we read the Bible, we find that God is love. If He showed His love to people whom the world rejected, surely He can show his love to us. If He loved the lepers, the tax collectors, and the harlots, surely He can love us. When we read the Bible, we find that God performs the seemingly impossible. He parted the Red Sea. He gave sight to the blind and hearing to the deaf. He raised the dead. If God performed miracles then, surely He can do the seemingly impossible in our lives.

Once I began reading my Bible again, my faith increased. God did a miracle in my life by taking what the world called a severe disability and allowing me to share Him through it.

Lord, You enable me to minister when the world would leave me to vegetate. Make me eager to read the Word to build my faith.

~Jason R. Mitchener

God Sees Us As Finished

"Being confident of this, that He who began a good work in you will carry it on to completion until the day of Christ Jesus," (Philippians 1:6).

I recently made a quilt for my five-month-old granddaughter, Hannah. As I began to plan the pattern and color scheme, I imagined the perfect quilt. I drew the pattern on paper, checking every dimension. Then I went shopping for the fabrics; I carefully selected each color and design for every piece of the quilt. In my planning, I constantly envisioned this quilt as finished. I was the only one who had a vision of what this finished project would look like. To others, it looked like a pile of different fabrics and a piece of paper with lines on it. But I saw it pieced together, quilted, and finished, with Hannah all snuggled up under it.

As I cut and pieced the fabrics together, I saw a thing of beauty begin to take place before my eyes. It wasn't perfect, but being the designer of the quilt, I saw the beauty and the love in the quilt, that no one else could see.

God is the same way; He sees us finished. He sees that completed work in each of us and knows in advance how every circumstance of our life forms us into the person He has designed us to be. Living with chronic illness and pain is part of the finishing process that God allows to take place. Everything we experience with chronic illness can make our character more refined and the beauty of the Lord more defined in us. Each one of those things, like every piece of Hannah's quilt, is pieced together in the fabric of our lives to make something beautiful.

Lord, I am Your workmanship, and You have a plan within Your creation of me. You envision me finished! Thank You, Lord God, that You don't give up on me and that You will see me through to a completion that glorifies You. Each day may the beauty of You be more defined in me. *~Patty Dahl*

Our Father Is Holding Our Hand

"Yet I am always with you. You hold me by my right hand," (Psalm 73:23).

My husband can hold my hands, but he is the only one. You see, he knows just how to be firm, yet gentle. He can help me out of a car without pulling my wrist too hard. He knows to use caution when he's helping me get my coat on. He knows when to offer his hand in assistance without squeezing too much. He understands, despite the pain that my wrists and hands feel, they long to be touched, to be held, to be warmed. He knows how to rub them gently when they are swollen and red. He gets me ice every evening to put on them. When they have been in casts, he has cut the food on my plate and has tied my shoes. Is there any doubt why I trust his touch?

Our Father has a similarly perfect touch, a gentle yet firm grasp on us. In Psalm 73:23, God assures us, "Yet I am always with you. You hold me by my right hand." The Psalmist admits that he could not be without God because God is always holding onto his right hand. He never leaves our side. He understands that we have bruises, soreness, and places where we hurt—in our hearts and in our bodies. But we trust that God knows precisely how to soothe all of our hurts. He knows how to hold our hand so that we can find comfort, assurance, and confidence. When we hold God's hand, we have His strength available to us. We find that all things are possible through Him. We may lead Him to some places that He knows we shouldn't be, but just as a parent holds on to the hand of a child who wants to be independent and walk away, God is our parent who says, "I will go the distance with you."

Lord, I may become lost or even tempted by life's dangers. I have scars from the pain of this world, but You tightly grasp my hand and will not let go. You know that I need Your guidance, Your strength, and Your comfort. *~Lisa Copen*

Avoiding Tipped Scales

"The Lord detests differing weights, and dishonest scales do not please Him," (Proverbs 20:23).

"Who else is on this scale with me?" I wanted to ask at the doctor's appointment; I cringed when the nurse announced a figure in her cheery voice, that I never thought I would hear. I told her I was wearing my ten-pound shoes.

Many of us struggle with our weight, whether it be too high or too low. Others of us may not deal with weight issues, but we all have "our issues," and the Lord knows that we need to face reality when it comes to these challenges. It's never easy to admit that we are not perfect. In reading a book about my personality, I was able to admit that I do have a hard time acknowledging that my way is not always best. Proverbs 20:12 says, "Ears that hear and eyes that see, the Lord has made them both." Frequently, we find it easy to use our ears and eyes to see the faults in others. We notice that our kids didn't pick up their dirty clothes. We observe that our spouse spent the entire night watching television while we folded laundry and did the dishes, even though we are the ill one.

"Watch out!" writes Barbara Johnson. "God is making you authentic. Real. Rubbing off your fake fur. Changing your outlook. Giving you new desires. Making you marvelous. Fulfilling what you were *created* for. He is making you the 'Queen or King of Quite a Lot,' enlightening you for kingdom work.... Be *brave*. Then braver still. Never resist His insistence on your perfection."[50]

God, it's easy to tip the scales in my direction and blame those around me for my dissatisfaction. My scales are dishonest, however, and they do not please You. While I may be able to justify all of the reasons I have a right to be frustrated, You know the truth and my lack of servanthood attitude. Help me face the truth and accept the reality so I can grow in character. *~Lisa Copen*

Searching For Strength

"To this end I labor, struggling with all his energy, which so powerfully works in me," (Colossians 1:29).

Corrie ten Boom once said, "Trying to do the Lord's work in your own strength is the most confusing, exhausting, and tedious of all work. But when you are filled with the Holy Spirit, then the ministry of Jesus just flows out of you."[51]

Before illness, I was considered physically strong for my size. I could carry two small children and manage to bring in a bag of groceries and the mail all at once without collapsing. I could clean the whole house, do all the running of errands around town, and manage supper, all without a nap. I even recall putting in a whole day's work without having to take medication. Though not so long ago, it sometimes seem as though it was a thousand years ago.

Pain and suffering now require me to seek help with the chores, take naps when I am weak, and seek medical attention when the symptoms of illness get the better of me. I feel so frail and useless. Those who have chronic pain can identify with my story. Some days I cannot find the strength to even get out of bed. Those are the days that I rely on Scriptures to see me through. This reminds me that I am loved and that somehow I can carry on.

Oh, what a promise, to hope in the Lord and to find strength in Him. I know that the Lord can renew my strength. Sometimes, although my physical strength may be weak, I can grow strong in my faith just by renewing the hope of our Lord's promises.

Oh, strengthen my faith that I may soar. Lord, with You I grow strong, weary no more. My spirit grows stronger, yet my body grows weak. I desire Your mercy. Your countenance, I will seek.

~Deborah Farmer

When Jesus Calls For You

"And after she had said this, she went back and called her sister Mary aside. 'The Teacher is here' she said, 'and is asking for you,'" (John 11:28).

Jesus did not forget Mary. In this true story that begins in tragedy and ends revealing the glory of God, Mary was grieving alone over the death of her brother. Martha had gone to meet Jesus as He made His way towards the tragic scene. Mary stayed behind. We are not told why. We can only imagine what she was feeling. She had a close relationship with Jesus. Why Jesus had not come earlier, to prevent the death of her brother, caused her confusion and probably a little bit of doubt as to whether He was as good, kind, and loving as she had believed.

He was. Jesus was carrying her close to His loving heart as He made His way toward the home of heartache and loss. Little did she know, a resurrection was soon to come! Are you confused and hurt, perhaps disappointed at God, for the circumstances that He has allowed in your life? While you're waiting, Jesus is preparing some secret joy for you that will be a special blessing from your hurt and pain! Jesus did not forget Mary. While she was weeping and in despair over the circumstances in her life, Jesus was making His way toward her to prove that He was the answer to her grief, sorrow, and her every need… and to perform a miracle.

He is making His way to you, Beloved, as you perhaps weep at the circumstances that He has allowed in your life. He will come to you; He will call for you, and He will turn your heartache into joy. You are His bride, His chosen one, and He ultimately only brings goodness and loving kindness into your life. Wait for Him. He is coming to you.

You say You will come again and receive me. I am listening for Your voice. I know You will call for me. *~Virginia Ganskie*

May We Always Respond With Compassion

"For I was hungry and you gave me something to eat.
I was thirsty and you gave me something to drink.
I was a stranger and you invited me in.
I needed clothes and you clothed me.
I was sick and you looked after me.
I was in prison and you came to visit me,"
(Matthew 25:35-36).

May we as God's people respond with compassion
to those around us in pain or distress.
May our words be a balm. . . a sweet, soothing comfort
on their spirits, weary for rest.
May our actions toward those who are suffering
reflect the kindness of Jesus, God's Son.
And may we notice the things the world overlooks
so we'll be known as the sensitive ones.
May God reveal the times we should be silent and listen,
or may He give us the right words to speak.
For it is His mission we long to fulfill
and His purpose and will that we seek.
May we cry out in prayer for those who need healing,
and may we remember them as we intercede.
May the Spirit of God join with us in prayer
with the wisdom to meet all of their needs.
We won't have all the answers to each other's problems
nor every situation will we understand.
But may we as God's children carry one another's burdens
and reach out with compassionate hands.

~Sheila Gosney

He Comes To Me

"If anyone loves Me. . . We will come to and make our home with him," (John 14:23).

The last time I went to church was over eight years ago. One of the hardest things about being confined to home is not being able to worship God with a congregation of people. It's not the same on my own, and in some ways I have felt cut off from the Lord's presence. I've had to work at remembering that He is always available and with me wherever I am.

In Revelation 3:20, He says, "If anyone hears My voice and opens the door, I will come in and eat with him and he with Me." He wants to meet with us in the very intimate areas of our lives. He makes His presence felt and communicates in so many little ways. I hear His voice more often than I did when I was healthier. I believe one of the blessings of chronic illness is that we have more time to spend with our Father. "Turn to me and be gracious to me, for I am lonely and afflicted," (Psalm 25:16) asks the Psalmist. I can use my lonely moments to draw close to God, as even Jesus did. "Jesus often withdrew to lonely places and prayed," (Luke 5:16).

We are blessed in New Zealand to have nationwide Christian radio, and I find that He often speaks to me through speakers or in the words of a song. Although the intended meaning is different, I have found one phrase of a song meaningful: "When I couldn't come to where He was, He came to me." Dear friend, if you're feeling cut off, know that He is just longing to come to you and meet with you just where you are, every moment of the day.

Loving Father, how privileged I am to have access to Your throne twenty-four hours a day; You are never too busy to listen or speak with me. When I can't get to places where Your people meet together, may I always be aware of Your loving presence close by, speaking quiet assurance into my life. *~Janice McLaren*

He Records Your Tears

"Record my lament; list my tears on Your scroll; are they not in Your record? Then my enemies will turn back, when I call for help. By this I will know that God is for me," (Psalm 56:8-10).

The darkness of night can be a frightening time for us who live with chronic illness or pain. When I am trying to go to sleep, the darkness brings on unwanted thoughts that I am able to avoid during the day because I am distracted by tasks. The darkness, however, contributes to my fears; I feel helpless, hopeless, despair, and doubt. Lying there, I can drown in my tears, wondering if I will make it another day.

Notice in the verse above, however, that it says our tears are recorded. God never sleeps, and He is always divinely present. When you wake up at 2:00 a.m. feeling panicked, as I do, He is there. When we call out to our Lord, He is always ready to come to our side. Then our enemies will turn back. Our fears, pains, and anxiety will all back off.

I have felt the darkness caving in on me in the night, and I have called out to Jesus to help me. And guess what? He always has. The morning always brings His new and fresh grace. He brings a new perspective.

Ken Gire, author, says, "Prayer is a cry from the bare spot in our lives, from the empty space, from the part of us that is missing. It is the wounded part seeking to be healed, the missing part seeking to be found, the now-dry clay of the sculpture seeking the hands that first touched it, first caressed it, first loved it."[52]

God, You are "for me" always. In the blackest black, Your eternal light will shine through. I will not be afraid to ask You to remember my tears, and to remember me. You know I love You, Lord. Every tear is lovingly recorded in the Book of Life. ~*Tina Nahid*

How Can I Live Like This?

"Though outwardly we are wasting away, yet inwardly we are being renewed day by day," (2 Corinthians 4:16).

A friend asked me the other day, "How can you say that your ministry is for people who *live* with chronic illness or pain? Most of us aren't living at all, we are merely just hanging on by a thread!" I answered her by saying, although I understood what she was saying, I felt that it is important that we each realize that we are a person with many facets, one of them being that we have a chronic illness. I dislike labeling myself as "chronically ill" because there is much more to me than just my illness. You are not your illness.

God has placed each of us here on earth for a purpose, and when we start to label ourselves as "chronically ill," we tend to forget that we are a child of God. Despite our illness, we still have a ministry that we are responsible for completing. Some of us are given a long life to complete this purpose. Others of us are not, and our time here on earth seems much too brief. Regardless of the length of our life, God wants us to have a life of depth. "Though outwardly we are wasting away, inwardly we are renewed day by day," (2 Corinthians 4:16).

How do we *live* with a chronic illness when we feel like we are stuck in survival mode? Keep spending time with the Father, surrendering your life to Him and being open to whatever ministry He desires for you. Abide in Him. Your wisdom and strength may be just what the Lord desires for you to, for example, witness to a nurse.

Lord, help my enduring patience be a legacy to those I love. This way, I can be reassured every day that I am not just someone who lives with chronic illness, I am someone who lives in the presence of God. Please take great delight in me and rejoice over me with Your singing, (Zephaniah 3:17b). *~Lisa Copen*

The Lord Is Fighting For Me

"The Lord will fight for you; you need only to be still," (Exodus 14:14).

"I had a friend once who had the same illness that you did," a woman at church explained to me. "He's dead now," (Gee, was that supposed to comfort me?) "Anyway, he got it because he was always just so busy. He couldn't sit still. He always had to be doing something. Do you think that could be your problem? I think that's probably why you got this disease! Maybe if you just slowed down…."

Well! She told me. I'll admit it: I am a busybody. I know, without doubt, that one of the ways the Lord wanted to use this illness was to see if He could slow me down and weed out some of the unimportant things out of my life. In an odd way, it worked, and I feel blessed that at the young age of twenty-four, upon diagnosis, I was able to learn what is truly important in this lifetime.

On the other hand, my illness hasn't slowed down my body as much as He may have hoped. I push through everything. I push to get out of bed. I push to get to the post office. I push to put away the groceries. And I grab any cart, counter, or vacuum cleaner nearby just to stand up at times. Driving home from the doctor's office the other day, with that overwhelming feeling of confusion about what my next step in treatment should be, I heard the Lord say, "Stop pushing!" *What? Stop? What use would I be to You then, Lord?* "Oh, my child. I don't need your help! Let me handle it. Sit still for a while and let Me fight this battle."

Father, it only makes sense. You already know the future! You know how best to fight my battle since You already know the outcome. Sometimes, the lesson I am meant to learn isn't in my doing, but in my sitting, my stillness. Oh, Lord, give me patience and strength to just sit. *~Lisa Copen*

The Gardener

"'I am the true vine, and My Father is the gardener. He cuts off every branch in Me that bears no fruit, while every branch that does bear fruit He prunes so that it will be even more fruitful… Remain in Me, and I will remain in you. No branch can bear fruit by itself, it must remain on the vine,'" (John 15:1-4).

My Father is a Gardener; His Son is the True Vine. I am grafted into Him, and all His power is mine. Without Him, I am nothing; but He has promised me, if I abide within the Vine, He will abide in me.

I had so many branches, abloom with flowers fair; I showed them to the Gardener, and hoped that He would share, my joy as I produced so many lovely things for Him. He looked at me with saddened eyes and began to shake each limb.

He took a knife, so sharp, so clean, and sheared off every flower. I cried as He destroyed the products of so many hours. I watched my leaves fall to the ground, along with all my tears. I saw them now for what they were—wasted days and years.

And when the Gardener finished, I looked with shame to see that ugly branches, naked limbs were all He left to me. The winter winds blew fierce on empty branches of my life; for I had known the full extent of the Gardener's knife.

I waited—seasons, days, and years—I do not know how long. But one day I began to feel faint birthings of a song; for there, on lonely branches, I gazed through tears to see the fruit restored. Yes, life had pushed through all the death in me.

I felt the power of the Vine flow sweetly through each limb; and then I knew the fruit would grow as I remained in Him. My Father is a Gardener; His Son is the True Vine. I am grafted into Him and all His power is mine.

~Connie Kennemer

Finding Joy In The Lord

"Shout for joy to the Lord, all the earth, burst into jubilant song with music; make music to the Lord with the harp, with the harp and the sound of singing, with trumpets and the blast of the ram's horn—shout for joy before the Lord, the King," (Psalm 98:4-6).

After several difficult days during the past week, the Lord has brought me through a storm of pain and a fight against depression. Today I am full of joy; His peace and love surround me. Joy has been missing for too long. I want to thank and praise Him with every fiber of my being! I want to respond like the Psalmist who urges us to acknowledge the joy of the Lord.

Many of you are probably thinking, "I can barely get out of bed and walk, much less have a 'joy fest' to the Lord." I challenge you today to make an attempt at being joyful. Picture the scene described in Psalm 98; hear the expressions of joy—jubilant songs, shouts of joy to the Lord, a harp playing beautiful songs of praise, accented by the sounds of trumpets and the ram's horn being blown enthusiastically as the crowd worships and exalts the Lord our God. Then keep this picture in your mind and heart. Recreate it and embellish upon it at any time, especially when you feel joyless or hopeless. Break away from your captivity of pain and chronic illness!

"The most valuable thing the Psalms do for me," wrote C. S. Lewis, "is to express the same delight in God which made David dance." "When the Lord brought back the captives to Zion we were like men who dreamed. '...The Lord has done great things for them.' The Lord has done great things for us, and we are filled with joy," (Psalm 126:1-3).

I will choose to be "joyful always; pray continually; give thanks in all circumstances, for this is God's will for [me] in Christ Jesus," (1 Thessalonians 5:16-18).

~Nancy Wilcox

You Are Wonderfully Made

"I praise You because I am fearfully and wonderfully made. Your works are wonderful. I know that full well. My frame was not hidden from You when I was made in the secret place. When I was woven together in the depths of the earth, Your eyes saw my unformed body. All the days ordained for me were written in Your Book before one of them came to be," (Psalm 139:14-16).

Wait a minute! I am what? Fearfully and wonderfully made? Lord, You are kidding, right? I mean, I have a body that does not work like it was designed to function. Are You sure You are talking to the right person? I read this Scripture and am stunned. We all know that we are loved, treasured, and led by Jesus. We praise Him for all He has done for us, but to actually thank Him for a body that has revolted against us – that's tough. Well, what does "wonderfully" mean anyway?

In *The New Strong's Complete Dictionary of Bible Words,* "wonderfully" is defined as, "to glean, to overdo, to be, make wonderful, miracle, and to distinguish." How can this define us? Because these words describe how the Father made us. Remember, we were made in His image, which is nothing but perfection. You were knit together in your mother's womb, and Jesus knew you before there was even conception. There has always been a plan for you, disability or not.

Do we actually have to thank Him for what we have? Honestly, I cannot look at my leg that is three times as large as it should be, filled with constant pain, and be grateful. I can, however, thank God for what having this condition has done for my life. I am not the same person that I was before, and I will never, ever go back. If you can't thank Him yet, that's okay. Just know that He loves you, there is a purpose, and never let go of God's Almighty hand.

"Who, O God, is like You? Though You have made me see troubles, many and bitter, You will restore my life again," (Psalm 71:19,20).

~Rebecca Koszalinski

A Note From An Angel

"For He will command His angels concerning you to guard you in all your ways; they will lift you up in their hands, so that you will not strike your foot against a stone," (Psalm 91:11,12).

I recently went to see my cardiologist for an echocardiogram. I have been doing poorly; one of my medications has been increased and decreased, leaving me in a state of breathlessness when walking more than fifty feet. Prior to my appointment, I went into the ladies' room to freshen up.

Taped to the mirror was a small piece of paper. Someone had typed a Scripture verse onto it and entitled it, "For You." The verse read: "I lift up my eyes to the hills. Where does my help come from? My help comes from the Lord, the Maker of heaven and earth," (Psalm 121:1,2). I was feeling alone and scared, and a blessed angel sent me this note. I quickly put it in my purse, and a calm peace seemed to envelop me. Someone was encouraging another daily, (Hebrews 3:13), and I was the blessed recipient.

In the midst of our pain and despair, know that God walks with you always. The Maker of heaven and earth is your help. All you need to do is to reach out and take a hold of His Hand. Let your prayer to God be: "I wait for the Lord, my soul waits, and in His Word I put my hope," (Psalm 130:5).

Author Andrew Murray wrote, "Let your faith in Christ be in the quiet confidence that He will every day and every moment keep you as the apple of His eye, keep you in perfect peace and in the sure experience of all the light and the strength you need."[53]

Lift my eyes to the hills of where You reside, O God, from where Your help comes. Place my hope in Your Word of love so that Your grace and mercy may bless me beyond measure. ~*Kay DeCarlo*

Expect Unexpected Blessings

"Then the Lord said, 'I will surely return to you about this time next year, and Sarah, your wife, will have a son.' Now Sarah was listening at the entrance to the tent, which was behind Him. Abraham and Sarah were already old and well advanced in years, and Sarah was past the age of childbearing," (Genesis 18:10,11).

There are moments in life that are etched in our memory. The day that my surgeon walked into the exam room, with a diagnosis finally in hand, is one of those moments. He merely asked me, "Do you have children?" "No," I replied, biting my lip to keep a hold of my emotions. Then he asked, "Did you want to have children?" At that moment, I knew that I was dealing with something serious. Due to the health issues and resulting disability, the medical professionals advised me that childbearing would be too risky. I was crushed, although I had not yet even found the man I was to marry and with whom I would pray to have a child.

On my wedding day, that same surgeon came through the receiving line and whispered in my ear, "Don't get pregnant." Months later, I called to tell him that I was pregnant. Most of all, however, I will always remember holding my healthy, normal baby boy in my arms, at my breast, reveling in the miracles God had displayed in my life.

Sarah laughed too. She looked at her aging body and found it impossible that God would use her for such a purpose. Abraham protested that he was also far too old, as Sarah stifled a giggle. God showed His mercy as He was scoffed at by two mere humans, who were so unaware of the bigger picture. He has the blueprint, and nothing that He has planned can be thwarted!

Though I have pain and illness, though my body has betrayed me and the medical profession has warned me of a bleak future, You, O God, will not be stopped! I know You, trust You, and believe You!

~Rebecca Koszalinski

Being With Jesus

"He appointed twelve... that they might be with Him," (Mark 3:14a,c).

Priceless, precious words these are to my soul: He appointed twelve, that they might be with Him. We who suffer with chronic pain often mourn as we see others go about their lives not tied down by pain or affliction. We may long for the days of the past when we could exercise or do anything we wanted, not hampered by a diseased body.

Often the only thing we can do on "bad pain days" is to be with Jesus. But of all our pursuits in life, this is the most fulfilling and joyful. Let us look at our situation through God's eyes. Mankind's highest calling is to be with God. It often takes pain and affliction to bring a soul close to Him. What special people we must be that God would choose us to hear His heartbeat for ourselves, and then to pass the knowledge of Him on to others.

"Now this is eternal life: that they may know You, the only one true God, and Jesus Christ, whom You have sent," (John 17:3). To know Him, we must spend time with Him. He wants to reveal Himself to us, and He desires for us to share our burdens, fears, hopes, and joys with Him. On our bad days, this may be all that we can do, but it is enough. "When you become consumed by God's call on your life," shares Charles Stanley, "everything will take on new meaning and significance. You will begin to see every facet of your life—including your pain—as a means through which God can work to bring others to Himself."[54]

God, You are enough. When I look at my situation, perplexity, fear, anger, or depression may set in; but when I look at it through Your eyes, I feel special and privileged. I am one of the ones that You have chosen to just sit at Your feet and learn of You, by You. How special I must be to You for You to choose me to be so close to Your Holy presence.

~Virginia Ganskie

Will God Let Me Complain?

"He will call upon me, and I will answer him; I will be with him in trouble, I will deliver him and honor him," (Psalm 91:15).

I can't imagine not being able to talk to Jesus freely about my aches and pains. It is such a comfort to know that God will always be there to listen. What a joy it is to know that God promises to be right beside me, even when I am complaining.

On the other hand, God can grow weary of our complaints if we make the choice to just walk in circles and moan about our circumstances. Friendship with God is the ability to be truly authentic, completely honest, without forgetting that we are in His Holy presence. I keep most of my discomforts to myself, because I know my friends would grow tired of my presence if I shared with them every ache that I had. When it comes to talking with Jesus, however, I just let it all out.

However, the God that says, "He will call upon me and I will answer him," is the same God that said, "How long will this wicked community grumble against me? I have heard the complaints of these grumbling Israelites," (Numbers 14:27).

We wrestle with mixed emotions, as did Job. One moment he was saying, "If I say, 'I will forget my complaint, I will change my expression, and smile,'" (Job 9:27). The next moment he said, "I loathe my very life; therefore I will give free rein to my complaint and speak out in the bitterness of my soul," (Job 10:1).

"You are forfeiting the grace that could help you through that trial by complaining about it," writes James MacDonald in *Lord, Change My Attitude*. "All the grace and strength you need to experience joy and victory is available to you."[55]

Lord, I never want to stop talking to You. Help me avoid getting on a soapbox, but help me get on my knees… You are Holy. I await Your response.
~Lisa Copen

It's in His Hands

"I did this so that you might know that I am the Lord your God," (Deuteronomy 29:6).

As a small child I favored the song, "He's Got the Whole World in His Hands." It was a reassuring thought that God had the whole world in His hands. My childlike faith did not know skepticism, and I lived in my little neighborhood where worries were few and peace was taken for granted. Then I grew up. Somehow, although I still wanted to believe that He had the whole world in His hands, the evening news didn't give the assurance I was searching for. If He *had* the whole world in His hands, why was He shaking us up like a two-year-old with a new snow globe? What was happening here?

Illness entering my life was like a snow globe being shaken until everything that was once clear became blurry and foggy. Life wasn't covered with a beautiful snow, but rather a half-inch of ashen flakes that seemed would never clear. In time, they did. Illness has refined my life. Illness has knocked out that which was unimportant; it has condensed it to what I can do at this moment. Like my grandmother before me, every time I commit to something, in my mind I am thinking, "Lord-willing." There is nothing that truly needs to be done if God does not provide the means to allow me to do it. "Now listen, you who say, 'Today or tomorrow we will go to this or that city, spend a year there, carry on business and make money.' Instead, you ought to say, 'If it is the Lord's will, we will live and do this or that,'" (James 4:13,15).

The snow in our snow globe will clear. It takes time. It's hard to be patient. Just as the flakes settle, it seems God is shaking it up again, making us wait even longer. Life feels like one snowstorm after another. It will. This isn't heaven.

Lord, help me to learn to enjoy the snow until one day You and I are walking the streets of gold together, hand in hand. You do have Your whole world in Your hands. ~*Lisa Copen*

Jesus Found Him

"Jesus heard that they had thrown him out, and when He found him..." (John 9:35a).

Jesus heard that the Pharisees had cast a man out of the synagogue, the same man that He had healed of his blindness; so He went looking for the man. Jesus understood the repercussions of being cast out of the house of worship. This man had already endured the accusations of bringing blindness upon himself by sinning, for that was the social belief of the day. He had likely endured much humiliation, and now he was cast out of the synagogue.

But Jesus searched for him, found him, and then revealed to him who He was. Imagine being blind all of your life, then to be healed, and one of the first faces that you see is the face of God! Dear one, perhaps you feel like a castoff today because of chronic pain or illness. Perhaps your spouse has told you that they would like a divorce. Or the "religious leaders" in the church have informed you that someone else will be doing the job that you thought would eventually be yours. Perhaps your family and friends rarely desire to spend time with you. There are many causes of feeling "castoff."

Know this: Of you feel like you have been castoff, Jesus wants to seek you out, just as He did the blind man over two thousand years ago. His Word to you today is: "I have loved you with an everlasting love; I have drawn you with loving-kindness," (Jeremiah 31:3). Precious one, Jesus is looking for you today. He wants to wrap His loving arms around you. He longs for you to share life together with Him in an ever more intimate way.

Lord, You say, "I myself will tend my sheep and have them lie down, [declares the Sovereign Lord]. I will search for the lost and bring back the strays. I will bind up the injured and strengthen the weak, but the sleek and the strong I will destroy. I will shepherd the flock with justice," (Ezekiel 34:15,16). *~Virginia Ganskie*

Finding A Joyful Life

"He seldom reflects on the days of his life, because God keeps him occupied with gladness of heart," (Ecclesiastes 5:20).

As I was coming up the road to my home today, I was overwhelmed with how much goodness God has given me in this life. Life is not easy. In fact, it is much more difficult than I'd ever imagined. It can become tempting to look around at the lives that others have and envy them. I sometimes envy their abilities. Other times I long for their innocence, of knowing life without health problems. But overall, I feel blessed and am grateful for what I have.

The other day a person quoted to me, "One who has his health has a joyful and abundant life." I smiled at him and said, "Sorry, but that's not true. I don't have my health, but I still have a joyful and abundant life." Our joy is not dependent on our health.

How is this? How are we able to respond with joy in the face of trials? It is only through the love and grace of God that we can find this joy. Ecclesiastes 5:20 says, "He seldom reflects on the days of his life, because God keeps him occupied with gladness of heart." If I were to sit and think about the challenges I face each day, the feeling of isolation a chronic illness can instill, the relationships that have not survived my illness, and the child I have not been given, I would quickly become downcast. "Pain is inevitable, but misery is optional," writes Tim Hansel. "We cannot avoid pain, but we can avoid joy. God has given us such immense freedom that He will allow us to be as miserable as we want to be."[56]

When I keep my focus on You, loving God, You fill my heart with a joy that I could never be given from this world. What delight You must feel when I become so preoccupied with You that I forget the world's standards that "one must have his health to live joyfully…"

~Lisa Copen

Remind Me

"So I will always remind you of these things, even though you know them and are firmly established in the truth you now have,"
(2 Peter 1:12).

Lord, when I am too weary to go on,
Remind me to rest in You.
When tears of sadness insist on flowing,
Remind me that one day all tears will be wiped away.

When pain and illness surround me,
Remind me that You understand
through suffering on Calvary.
When those I love are far away and I cannot be with them,
Remind me that You, are there and let them know I care.

When I've lost my joy and happiness,
Lord, let me remember past joys and
that future joys are coming.
When I am broken and useless and want to go Home,
Remind me that time is in Your hands.

When I feel so alone and lost,
Remind me that You have promised
never to leave me nor forsake me.
When fear and panic encompass me
and I don't even know why,
Remind me that "Greater is He that
is in you than he that is in the world."

When I am not all that I should be,
Lord, remind me that I am Your child
and to behave as such.
When I become discouraged because
of things I am no longer able to do,
Remind me that there are others in
the same situation, and worse.

When the dark loneliness surrounds me,
Lord, thank You for reminding others to send a note.
Lord, above all,
never let me forget what You suffered for me.
Help me to get my mind off of me
and onto others, as You would have me do.

Help me, Lord, to bring happiness and
joy to others. That is my desire.
Lord, remind me of sunshine and
flowers and things I don't always see.

Lord, remind me that a better day is coming.

~Jeanie Hutton

Take Courage!

"Jesus went out to them, walking on the lake. When the disciples saw Him walking on the lake, they were terrified. 'It's a ghost,' they said, and cried out in fear. But Jesus immediately said to them: 'Take courage! It is I. Don't be afraid,'" (Matthew 14:25-27).

My husband and I recently rescued a Brittany spaniel. We found "Daphne" on an Internet rescue web site. We have been enjoying her many sweet antics and playful ways, but I recently began to notice that she was having nightmares. My sweet dog, I believe, has post-traumatic stress, just as I. She was running and crying in the middle of the night. Distressed to see her like this, I adjusted my covers at the end of the bed and held her close to me, gently whispering, "Everything is okay. You are safe. Mommy and Daddy are here."

How many times do we suffer within a haven of fear, setting up walls around us for protection from the outside? I have done this on many occasions, yet, even in my fear, I seem to always run to the feet of my Lord and Savior, Jesus. I know that there is no comfort like that which He can provide. How do I know this? By experience. Jesus has said, "All authority in heaven and on earth has been given to Me," (Matthew 28:18). If this is so, some of you may ask, *Why do I have to suffer so?* Do you forget that our Savior has nail marks indented in His hands? Suffering is a part of life.

"When you and I hurt deeply, what we really need is not an explanation from God but a revelation of God," says author Warren W. Wiersbe. "We need to see how great God is; we need to recover our lost perspective on life. Things get out of proportion when we are suffering, and it takes a vision of something bigger than ourselves to get life's dimensions adjusted again."[57] In our distress remember we have Jesus, a redemptive Savior, to intercede on our behalf.

"'And surely [You are] with [me] always, to the very end of the age,'" (Matthew 28:20). ~*Kay DeCarlo*

Refuse To Be Discouraged

"Where can we go? Our brothers have made us lose heart. They say, `The people are stronger and taller than we are; the cities are large, with walls up to the sky'" (Deuteronomy 1:28).

David Ring was born with cerebral palsy and was orphaned at an early age. Years later, he gave his life to Christ, feeling the call to preach. People tried to discourage him, saying his slurred speech would never allow him to preach. David ignored them, becoming a nationally known preacher who speaks to over a hundred thousand people a year. When speaking about the obstacles he overcame, David asks his audience, "I have cerebral palsy. What's your problem?"

My father was also disabled. He spoke across the country at conferences and hospitals. He once said, "Nature disables us, but we allow people to handicap us." Often, we allow people to handicap us by letting them discourage us. This is exactly what happened to the Israelites. God wanted them to enter the Promised Land, but they listened to a few men who said it couldn't be done. God planned to give them the power to defeat the enemy, but the Israelites gave in to discouragement and ended up wandering the wilderness for forty years. Imagine if more people had given in to discouragement? "Simon Peter, stop that preaching! You're just a fisherman!" "Helen Keller, you're blind and deaf. You have no business writing!" "Abraham Lincoln, you've lost more political races than you've won. Quit trying to run for president!"

When God shows you the path He desires for you to travel, don't let others discourage you, even when the circumstances don't appear to be in your favor. Keep ministering for Jesus, regardless of others' skepticism.

God, give me the strength to accomplish Your purpose. When others say, "You can't," I will tell them, "In Christ, I can." Help me cling to Your words, "'With man this is impossible, but not with God; all things are possible with God,'"(Mark 10:27). *~Jason R. Mitchener*

It's Not About Me

"Father, if You are willing, take this cup from Me; yet not My will, but Yours be done," (Luke 22:42).

My husband and I and two dear friends gathered around a piano on a church stage as it neared midnight. Melanie had just lost her spouse, our precious friend; we gathered in the church where he had fallen from heart failure as he led worship days before. Tears fell, words were spoken, hugs were given generously, and my husband and Mel sat at the piano, allowing it to express emotions that were too raw to discuss.

Karen spoke of her pending test results to see if she would someday lose her voice, that which she valued so much as a vocalist. Mel raised her hands during worship, surrendering over the loss of her sweet husband. They both said, "It's not about me; it's about Him." The conversation turned toward my illness and a possible treatment one had heard of. I thanked them and said, "But it's not about me." They deeply wanted to fix the pain. I understand the feeling of wanting to fix it, but like both of their trials, it is in God's hands.

A tender subject turned into a God-filled moment, however. Despite my lack of ability to comprehend Mel's deep pain, God somehow provided a kind of reassurance to her, through my illness, that despite her pain, someday it will be okay. It's not about us. It's not about me. This book is not about our writers. We are simply broken vessels, allowing God to fill a few pores in order to allow us to carry His message, even if only a short distance, to someone who is hurting. To live as Jesus is to say, *Please, Lord, isn't there another way?* and then in the same breath say, *It's not about me. Thy will be done.*

Lord, the surrender is painful, but it is oh, so sweet. No cure will ever bring us closer to Your presence than the sound of those simple words, "It's not about me, Jesus. It's about You." *~Lisa Copen*

Concluding Thoughts

Wait! Before you finish this book, I can't let you close it without asking a very important question. Do you know the Lord Jesus as your Savior? I'm not asking, "Are you a Christian, do you go to church, or were you baptized?" I mean do you have a *personal relationship* with the Lord and Savior, the one whom the writers share about within these pages?

No one knows why illness came crashing uninvited into your life—not your spouse, not your pastor, not your parent, not your best friend. There are many reasons why God calls us to suffer. What we do know is that the reason for the affliction, or "the thorn," is fully and completely within God's knowledge alone. God says, "For My thoughts are not your thoughts, neither are your ways My ways," (Isaiah 55:8).

Perhaps, you are living with shame because you believe that your past actions could be a reason that God has allowed you to have this illness. Maybe you've tried to be a "good person," but "friends" have pointed out that the sin in your life is causing you to suffer and it is your fault. Perhaps when you reflect back on the past few years, like the African Proverb says, you think, "I have come a long way; the journey has exhausted me." The journey *will* exhaust you; you cannot do this alone.

While I do believe that God can use our illnesses to get our attention, I don't believe that He takes pleasure in seeing us hurt; even our pain is part of our growing process. Charles Swindoll acknowledges, "The path of obedience is marked by times of suffering and loss. When you suffer and when you lose, it does not mean... it's not tantamount to saying you are in disobedience. It might mean you're right in the center of His will."[58]

Let's take a brief look at some of the issues we run into if we believe that illness is a result of sin.

Isaiah 57:18 says, "I have seen his ways, but I will heal him; I will guide him and restore comfort to him." God saw one man's sin and restored comfort anyway. After Jesus healed another man by the pools, He told him, "Stop sinning or something worse may happen to you," (John 5:14). The man had been sinning, but Jesus chose to approach the man and offer him healing despite the sin.

God is not out to trick us into coming to Him. We live in a world that is full of sin, and we need God. It's as simple as that. "Seek the Lord while He may be found; call on Him while He is near," says Isaiah 55:7. While God is always near to us, I believe that the more we turn away from Him and say, "I can do this on my own. I don't need any help. I'm angry with God right now," the easier it becomes to keep pushing God away. And we push and we push, and then we wonder why we feel so alone, so empty, and so hopeless.

God has a purpose for this adversity in your life. Go ahead, get mad, cry out to God, ask Him questions. But then listen for His answers. Read the Psalms, read Job, read the book of John. There is no emotion that you are feeling that is not described within the pages of the Bible. I hope that this devotional book will become worn well, with pages folded over, notes on the edge of the writings, and even some passages highlighted. More than anything, however, I pray that it will cause you to look at a Scripture in a different light, and focus on it and what it means in your life. I hope you will be astonished at how specifically God uses Scriptures to describe not only our pain, but also our hope. I hope *Mosaic Moments* makes you want to get out your Bible and look up a Scripture that was referenced and then read a little further. There is power in His Word, power that paperback books will not fulfill in your life.

Despite the amazing ways that God has used my illness to reach out to others, I have moments when I wish He could have given me a ministry that didn't hurt so badly. We're human. Life is hard, and pain is not fun! It postpones plans and rocks relationships. It even disintegrates some dreams. Despite the fact that the writers and I may sound like we have it all together, we still go to sleep many nights with tearstains on our pillows. The difference is that we feel comforted by our Lord when we cry. Those without Him only feel lonely.

If you're tired of feeling lonely, if you're tired of wondering what your purpose is, if you're just plain sick and tired of being sick and tired, accepting the Lord as your Savior and friend is the answer. It doesn't mean your circumstances will change; it does mean your ability to live life will be whole, fulfilled, and you will be strengthened, even in the trials. You'll be given peace in the midst of chaos, joy in the midst of sorrow. You'll wonder how you ever survived before you knew God. With all this pain, why would you consider turning down the strength and joy given freely by the Creator of the universe? The Lord offers it all to you through Him. You just have to accept His gift.

Perhaps you are one who accepted Christ into your life some time ago, but now that you are living with daily pain, God has taken the brunt of the anger and emotional turmoil that you are experiencing. You may even have friends that condone this line of thought. Job's own wife advised him, "Are you still holding on to your integrity? Curse God and die!" (Job 2:9). But you know how hard it is to live without God. . . You want Him back.

It's never too late to start again and ask God into your life. Ask Him to take control of it, as you know you are unable to control it. Ask God to hold you close in His arms, tight enough that you can actually feel the Holy Spirit warming up your soul. I'm a do-it-myself, independent, know-it-all kind of girl, so I understand struggling with letting go and giving it over to God. But I must. Holding onto my life myself is even more painful and disheartening than humbling myself to say, *Lord, I need You, O, I need You.*

It's easy. Let's walk through it together. . . .

Admit that you are a sinner. Guess what? Nobody is perfect. Even though we try to be "good" and do the right thing, we still fall short. No one is exempt, "for all have sinned and [fallen] short of the glory of God," (Romans 3:23). Go ahead and tell God, "I've messed up. I've mucked up my life, and I need You to take it over. I can't do this by myself. I know I've sinned. I know I've done things that are not pleasing to You, but I want to change. I may not understand why You accept me just as I am, but I believe that You do. God, the Bible says that You tell me, "'Come now, let us reason together… though your sins are like scarlet, they shall be white as snow; though they are red as crimson, they shall be like wool,'" (Isaiah 1:18). I am Yours.

Accept that Jesus Christ is the Son of God and that He paid the price of your sin so that you may have eternal life. God's Word says, "God demonstrates His own love for us in this: While we were still sinners, Christ died for us," (Romans 5:8). All you have to do is accept this. Nothing you do will ever be enough. That's good news for us chronically ill folks! Our works don't matter. We receive Christ through faith. "For it is by grace you have been saved, through faith—and this not from yourselves, it is the gift of God—not by works, so that no one can boast," (Ephesians 2:8-9).

Call out to God your desire. "If you confess with your mouth, 'Jesus is Lord,' and believe in your heart that God raised Him from the dead, you will be saved," (Romans 10:9). Talk to Him. Give Him your heart. Yes, God is Holy, but He is also called Abba, which means He is your daddy. You can pour out your feelings of loneliness and the turmoil of feeling like no one understands what you are going through. Share with Him your deepest fears that you don't want to admit to anyone else. Even if it feels uncomfortable, just say, "Lord, I don't know what I am doing, but I am trusting You to show me who You are. I want to know You. I can't do this life alone another minute."

I encourage you to seek out someone and tell him or her about your decision today. Call a local church or call Rest Ministries and say, "I just gave my heart to the Lord. Now what?" If you don't have a Bible or are just looking for a personal one, contact us at the Rest Ministries web site and we will let you know what Bible is currently in print that may best meet your needs.

Romans 9:21 says, "Does not the potter have the right to make out of the same lump of clay some pottery for noble purposes and some for common use?" Illness hurts. Being molded into something noble is not an easy process. But grasp onto the joy that your common-use life is in the past. The potter is now making you into something noble. "But I was happy common," you may cry. It's true; but God will give you more than you can ask or imagine only through this journey. Psalm 68:6a, says, "God sets the lonely in families." Welcome to our family.

~May God bless you with a thirst for Him,

Lisa

About Rest Ministries

Rest Ministries is a Christian organization for people who live with chronic illness or pain. There are a variety of ways to connect with others through our programs and resources. The web site, www.restministries.org, offers over 300 pages of information for your benefit. For example, sign up to receive more of these daily devotionals that are sent out each morning for free online. Look for a pen pal, read articles from our newsletter, or join a discussion group to be encouraged daily.

Rest Ministries also has a small group program called HopeKeepers®. There are a few hundred HopeKeepers groups across the United States and beyond. Visit our web site or call us to receive an information packet on starting a HopeKeepers group for your church or neighborhood.

Rest Ministries the sponsor of *National Invisible Chronic Illness Awareness Week,* held annually in September. Visit www.invisibleillness.com for more information. And we have a weekly radio program called Hope Endures. See www.myhopeendures.com for scheduling.

Thank you for the purchase of this book. It assists us in supporting the financial needs of the organization so that we can continue to reach over 50,000 people per month.

Rest Ministries' Contact Information:
Phone: 888-751-7378 or 858-486-4685
Web Site: www.restministries.org
Address: P.O. Box 502928, San Diego, CA 92150
* *Submissions of 350-word devotionals for future devotional books can be sent to:* rest@restministries.org *with the subject "More Mosaic Moments."*

Did you enjoy this book? We'd love to hear from you, and please let us know if we can share your comments/reviews with others.

Get The Online Devotionals

To sign up for Rest Ministries daily devotionals, go to: www.chronicillnessdevotionals.com

You can even include code to put them on your own web site and have them automatically update each morning.

If you are not on the Internet, but you do have an email program, you are also able to participate. Just send a blank email to chronicpaindevotional-subscribe@yahoogroups.com

About The Contributors

PATRICIA ARMSTRONG is a retired elementary schoolteacher who lives in Virginia Beach, Virginia, with her husband, Richard. Patricia suffers with constant pain from a nerve disease but has found purpose in her pain as it has brought her closer to the Lord and made her more understanding and supportive of others who are suffering. She knows God will never give us more than we can bear.

HOLLY BAKER lives in Dallas, Texas, with her husband and three teenagers and an Australian shepherd companion dog. Although she has had multiple sclerosis for twenty-one years and is in an electric wheelchair, she continues to enjoy her family, friends, church, and going practically anywhere. God has given her a bright hope, a glorious future, and the power to live this life.

PEGGIE BOHANON is a Christian homemaker, freelance writer and editor, and web master of *Peggie's Place,* (www.peggiesplace.com), known as "the most fun Christian home on the Web!" She has written for various publications and curriculum, and has been a guest on *Focus on the Family, Christian Computing Live,* and Moody Broadcasting Network. Peggie and her husband, Dr. Joseph Bohanon, an organic chemistry professor at Evangel University, reside in Springfield, Missouri; they have two teenage sons.

FIONA BURROWS is single and lives in Melbourne, Australia. She writes, when she can, to express her feelings and some of the things she has learned. She has chronic back pain but knows that only by relying on God and His strength can she face each new day and the challenges in it.

RON CAMERON lives in Sydney, Australia, with his wife, Jane. They have two adult children, one married and one still living at home. Ron lives with Parkinson's disease and has retired from full-time employment. He is involved with the work of his local church and enjoys various aspects of computing.

LISA COPEN is the founder of Rest Ministries, a Christian organization that serves people who live with chronic illness or pain (www.restministries.org). She is the author of various chronic illness Bible studies, books and has been published in magazines, and the anthology, *God Allows U-Turns: A Woman's Journey*. She's lived with rheumatoid arthritis since the age of twenty-four, diagnosed in '93, and also fibromyalgia. She does web design and Internet marketing for small businesses. She lives in San Diego, California, with her husband, Joel, where they await to adopt a child.

MARY LOU CORNISH admits to having been a lukewarm Christian for many years. Three car accidents changed that. Their legacy of pain and disability have drawn her into a deep, intimate relationship with the Lord, attesting to the fact that all things do indeed work together for good for those who love God and are called according to His purpose.

KAY DeCARLO is the devotional coordinator for Rest Ministries. She lives with her husband and two sweet dogs, Daphne and Greta, in New England. Kay, a survivor of Hodgkin's Disease and other life traumas, has never lost sight of God's mercy and grace. Kay struggles with dilated cardiomyopathy, a heart disease that affects the pumping chambers of her heart, bipolar disorder, depression and, anxiety. She prays daily to be an instrument by which God can use her to encourage and strengthen others. Kay prays for 2 Corinthians 1:3,5 to be the theme of her life.

PATTI DAHL lives in Southern California with her husband, Bob. She is a Bible teacher and one day would like to write a devotional or stories about her experiences living with multiple chronic illnesses and pain. It is her heart's desire to bring hope and encouragement to those who are lonely, discouraged, and hurting.

KARLTON DOUGLAS lives in Ohio with his wife and daughter. He enjoys reading and writing. He is a columnist for the *Appalachian Quarterly Magazine*, and his writing has been featured within numerous Internet web sites and newsletters. He is the author of *Chronic Illness: Living With A Thorn*, and a fictional book, *Griffin Island*. Karlton has endured the affliction chronic fatigue syndrome for more than a decade; he's found that God is faithful and His grace is sufficient.

NORMA ECKBLAD dedicated her life fully to the Lord at the age of fifteen and married Michael when she was eighteen; they have been married twenty-seven years. She was diagnosed with stage III Non-Hodgkin's Lymphoma in February 2002. She is now in remission. They have four grown children, who all were home to lovingly take care of her during her cancer battle.

ERICA FARAONE, author, singer, and speaker, loves to point people to Jesus. Erica lives in Whitefish, Montana, with her wonderful husband, Scott. At 33, Erica is recovering from twelve years of fibromyalgia and gives the Lord great praise for the gradual healing work He's done, and is still doing, in her body.

DEBORAH FARMER lives with her husband and two teenagers in Bunn, North Carolina. A homeschool mom, Deborah suffers from fibromyalgia and other chronic conditions. Having had several poems published when she was younger, Deborah went on to write a number of gospel songs before writing devotionals of encouragement for others who are in pain.

JUDY GANN lives in Lakewood, Washington, and is a freelance writer and children's librarian. She has fibromyalgia and mixed connective tissue disorder. Judy is in the process of writing a devotional book for those who are ill. Her writing credits include a true story in *Comfort for the Grieving Heart,* by Margolyn Woods, and two prayers in *Prayers for Troubled Times,* by Jeannie St. John Taylor.

VIRGINIA GANSKIE, her husband, Ken and two cats live in lovely Grass Valley, California. She suffers from chronic back and leg pain. These devotionals are a result of her never-ending search to know God and His beautiful character. Her desire is that, whether through her life or through her writings, people would come to know Jesus on a more personal level.

SHEILA GOSNEY, thirty-eight, is a wife and mother to three sons. Born and raised in Hannibal, Missouri, Sheila writes poems on many different topics, but her specialty is poems written on the subject of pain and suffering, from her own personal experiences with God. Sheila lives with Sjogren's disease and is the mother of a son with autism. Tasting God's healing, but also seeing where He has allowed suffering to continue, fully convinced her that God can be glorified in either situation.

JEANIE HUTTON lives in Vienna, West Virginia, with her pastor husband Gene. She is the mother of six, grandmother of soon to be thirteen and great grandmother of one. She does not consider herself a writer nor a poet, but loves putting thoughts into writing. Jeanie has post-polio syndrome and is in a wheelchair most of the time. God has made the journey with PPS bearable with His Presence. To see more of her writings, visit her page at www.christianpoetry.org/hutton.html

CONNIE KENNEMER is a fifty-year-old woman who is learning to steward weakness. Diagnosed with multiple sclerosis in 1994, she lives with limitations that change daily. Connie is a writer, speaker, recording artist, wife, mother and prayer warrior. She and her husband, Rex, serve with Church Resource Ministries (crmnet.org), developing leaders for the church.

REBECCA KOSZALINSKI is a R.N. and graduate of the University of Wisconsin-Oshkosh College of nursing. She works as an R.N. Recruiter and lives daily with pain and disability caused by severe lymphedema. She has also experimented with wheelchair racing and recently won her first 5K race. Becky is also a wife and mother and gives thanks to Jesus Christ, her Lord and Savior for all the gifts in her life.

JANICE McLAREN is sixty, a mother of four, and a grandmother who lives alone in Oamaru, New Zealand. She's had ME (chronic fatigue syndrome) since 1984, and has been virtually housebound since 1994, much of this time confined to bed. Writing is a very recent venture. Thankful for God's wonderful family, she looks to the future with hope in Christ Jesus.

JASON R. MITCHENER was born with a rare neuromuscular disease that now confines him to an electric wheelchair and requires him to use a ventilator to breathe. His body may be confined, but his spirit soars free. His song lyrics and devotional writing inspire and encourage Christians to draw closer to God. Visit his web site at www.JasonMitchener.com.

TINA NAHID, thirty, is a stay-at-home mother and wife in Hopkinsville, Kentucky. She received her B.A. and M.A. in English. She has suffered much physically, but claims her healing through Jesus Christ. She enjoys writing devotionals, reading God's Word and other inspirational books, spending time with family, serving her church, hiking, and living for the Lord.

ELLIE O'STEEN, L.M.T. has lived with chronic pain conditions, fibromyalgia, arthritis, and asthma for over twenty-five years. Ellie has been a practicing Licensed Massage Therapist since 1984 and has worked in varied medical clinics. She now practices privately in Auburn, AL. She and her husband, Glynn, have been married thirty-five years and have one son. They raise two rescued greyhounds. Her favorite verse is Philippians 1:6.

MARY ANN REDONDO was born with a disorder that is diagnosed as neurofibromatosis (NF). Contrary to this disorder, it does not hold her back in her ministry to others who need love and encouragement from the Lord God. Her goal in this life is to minister the love of the Lord God to the hearts of people who are chronically ill. She has learned that there is more to her than the package she comes in, and she looks at her life as a gift from God.

ROXANNE M. SMITH has had severe low back pain from degenerative disk disease for thirteen years. Her disk problems force her to spend most of her time lying down, despite several surgeries and many other medical treatments. She is married to Andy, and they have a son, Jakob, who is six years old. She has written several articles for Lutheran magazines and Rest Ministries on coping with a disability. She is currently editing a newsletter from her home for a local children's ministry.

SHERYL SMITH, fifty-three, has been married thirty-two years to a supportive husband; they have two children and two grandchildren. She has chronic myofascial pain and high blood pressure that is being treated fairly successfully. She has had digital photos published and participates in the Kairos prison ministry that takes retreat weekends into medium/maximum security prisons. Her personal life mission statement is: "I will serve the Lord to the best of my understanding with all I have and am, in whatever state as He wills and directs."

NANCY WILCOX is a retired schoolteacher who lives in Concord, North Carolina, with her husband Ronald. She enjoys reading, writing, doing needlework and crafts, camping, singing in her church choir, and being a grandmother. Nancy lives with several chronic illnesses and serves as a HopeKeepers group leader.

Share Mosaic moments

Rest Ministries' desire is to reach out to those that are hurting from the thorn of chronic illness. We wish to offer the gift of an understanding friend for the journey, sharing God's unconditional love.

You can share this hope with others by making a donation to Rest Ministries, and a Mosaic Moments *book will be sent to a place where people are hurting. A sticker will be in the book that says,* "This book was donated by a friend who wishes to provide hope on the illness journey."

For each $6 you donate, a book will be sent to a nursing home, a prison, a retirement center, a hospital, hospice, a church ministry to the homebound, a disability ministry, or other places. You can specify a place if you wish.

Please send the following to Rest Ministries, Attn. Mosaic Moments Gift, P.O. Box 502928, San Diego, CA 92150:

- ❖ *Your payment information (a check made payable to Rest Ministries, or Visa/MC #, expiration date).*
- ❖ *Your contact information. We will send you a receipt. Your gift is tax-deductible.*
- ❖ *You can specify which organization/company you wish the book to be sent to with an address. If a place is not specified, it will go to a needy organization as listed above.*

Thank you for making a difference!

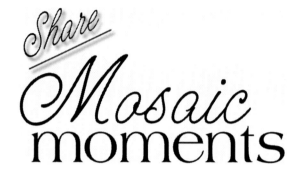

Notes

[1] Rev. Ken Hutcherson, former Seattle Seahawks linebacker, Pastor at Antioch Bible Church, Redmond, WA. Permission granted via C. Blazer.
[2] Presentation at Christian Council on Persons with Disabilities annual conference, 2001, Fullerton, CA.
[3] Deyneka, Peter & Anita, "Salvation and Suffering: The Church of the Soviet Union, *Christianity Today,* 16 July 1982, p. 19-21.
[4] Hansel, Tim. *You Gotta Keep Dancin'*. (David C. Cook Publishing, ©1985), p. 124.
[5] Wales, Susan, *Standing on the Promises*. (Multnomah Publishers, ©2001 Susan Huey Wales), p. 177
[6] Hansel, Tim. *You Gotta Keep Dancin'*. (David C. Cook Publishing, ©1985). p. 39.
[7] Frank, Anne. *The Diary of Anne Frank,* (Prentice Hall ©1993).
[8] Yancey, Philip. *Where is God When it Hurts* (Zondervan Publishing House, October 1, 2001).
[9] Lewis, C.S. *Mere Christianity: Comprising the Case for Christianity, Christian Behavior, and Beyond Personality (C.S. Lewis Classics),* (Touchstone Books, June 1996).
[10] Pepys, Samuel, *Pepy's Diary*: (1633 – 1703).
[11] Mayhall, Carole, *Lord of My Rocking Boat* (Colorado Springs: NavPress, 1981).
[12] *The Encouragement Bible*. (Zondervan Publishing House, March 1, 2001) p. 1349.
[13] General quote from various web sites, including "A Walk With God" web site, www.awalkwithgod.com
[14] Sultanoff, Steven M., Ph.D. "Examining the Research in the Therapeutic Benefits of Humor and Laughter" (©1999). www.humormatters.com.
[15] Cooper, Desiree, Free Press Columnist, *Detroit Free Press*. "Funny thing: Group Guffaws are Healthy." May 21, 2002.
[16] Chambers, Oswald. Daily Christian Quote, psalm121.ca/dcq.html.
[1717] Angelou, Maya, *Life Mosaic* by Hallmark, © 2001 M. Angelou & Hallmark Cards, Inc. Kansas City, MO 64141.
[18] Johnson, Samuel. Daily Christian Quote, psalm121.ca/dcq.html.
[19] Swindoll, Charles R., *Strengthening Your Grip*. (©1982 W Publishing Group (formerly Word, Inc.), Nashville, TN. Used by permission).
[20] Novotni, Michele and Randy Petersen, Angry with God; (NavPress, © 2001). p. 87.
[21] Daily Christian Quote Index at psalm121.ca/dcqelliot.html. Visit her web site *Gateway to Joy* at www.backtothebible.org/gateway/.
[22] *Pass It On*. Kurt Kaiser © 1969 by: Lexicon Music, Inc.
[23] Motivating Moments Inspirational Quotes, www.motivateus.com.
[24] Littleton, Mark, *The Storm Within* (Tyndale House Publishers, 1993). p. 89.
[25] Reported from various sources, but also noted that it may be an urban myth.
[26] *Christian Quote Daily*, Swan Lake Communications www.timothyreport.homestead.com/CQDaily.html.
[27] Author unknown.
[28] Mitchell, Margaret, *Gone with the Wind*. (Scribner Reprint edition, May 1996).
[29] *Christian Quote Daily*, Swan Lake Communications.www.timothyreport.homestead.com/CQDaily.html.
[30] *Merriam-Webster's Collegiate* 2002. (Merriam-Webster, Inc., 10th Index Edition, 1998).

[31] As heard on *Turning Point* radio show of Dr. David Jeremiah, Summer 2002, www.turningpointradio.org/radio.html
[32] Bond Stockdale, James. *A Vietnam Experience: Ten Years of Reflection* (Hoover Institution Press, Nov. 1984).
[33] Jowett, John Henry (1817-1893) -Edythe Draper, *Draper's Book of Quotations for the Christian World* (Wheaton: Tyndale House Publishers, Inc., 1992).
[34] *Women's Devotional Bible, NIV,* (Zondervan, 1990), p. 962.
[35] Littleton, Mark, *The Storm Within* (Tyndale House Publishers, 1993). p. 42.
[36] Lewis, C.S., *The Problem of Pain* (Harper San Francisco, February 5, 2001).
[37] Nightingale, Florence. *Notes on Nursing: What It Is and What It Is Not.* (1860). *Notes on Nursing: What It Is and What It Is Not Commemorative Edition.* (Lippincott Williams & Wilkins Publishers, December 1992).
[38] Ten Boom, Corrie. Corrie ten Boom Museum, www.corrietenboom.com.
[39] Lewis, C.S. *The Weight of Glory.* (Harper San Francisco, reprint March 20, 2001).
[40] Murray, Andrew, *Andrew Murray on Prayer.* (Whitaker House, 1998), pp. 18, 19.
[41] *From a Distance,* Written by Julie Gold. ©
[42] Yancey, Philip, *Where is God When it Hurts* (Zondervan Publishing House, October 1, 2001), p. 256.
[43] *The Encouragement Bible.* (Zondervan Publishing House, March 1, 2001) p. 540.
[44] Murray, Andrew. *Andrew Murray on Prayer: Abide in Christ,* (Whitaker House, 1998).
[45] Schuller, Robert H. *Tough Times Never Last, But Tough People Do!* Bantam, 1984) p. 64,65.
[46] Ten Boom, Corrie. Corrie ten Boom Museum, www.corrietenboom.com.
[47] Wright, H. Norman. Original source unknown. Reprinted from quote dataase from Zchurch, www.zchurch.com/dailymessage
[48] *Merriam-Webster's Collegiate,* 2002 (Merriam-Webster, Inc., 10th Index Edition, 1998).
[49] Elisabeth Elliot, Reprinted from *CQDaily Archives*: January 2000. www.timothyreport.homestead.com.
[50] Johnson, Barbara, quote database.
[51] ten Boom, Corrie. Corrie ten Boom Museum, www.corrietenboom.com.
[52] *Christian Quote Daily,* Swan Lake Communications www.timothyreport.homestead.com
[53] Murray, Andrew, *Andrew Murray on Prayer,* (Whitaker House, 1998).
[54]
[55] MacDonald, James. *Lord, Change My Attitude Before It's Too Late.* (Moody Press, 2001), p. 37.
[56] Hansel, Tim. *You Gotta Keep Dancin',* (David C. Cook Publishing, ©1985), p. 55.
[57] Adiar, James. *Be Quoted From A to Z* with Warren W. Wiersbe (Baker Books, April 2000).
[58] "Growing Through Loss," a sermon by Charles R. Swindoll, copyright 1997; tape number GRP-2B. Reprinted by permission of Insight for Living, Plano, TX 75026.

Ordering Information

[Quant]
_____ *Mosaic Moments* $14.00
_____ *Why Can't I Make People Understand?* $12.00
_____ *Beyond Casserolse: 505 Ways to Encourage a Chronically Ill Friend* .... $7.00 each or 3 for $15
_____ *A Woman's Health Resource Journal* $28.95
_____ *So You Want to Start a Chronic Illness/Pain Ministry: 10 Essentials For Making it Work* $15.00

Bible Studies
_____ *When Chronic Illness Enters Your Life (5 lessons)* $6.50
_____ *Learning to Live with Chronic Illness (5 lessons)* $6.50

❑ I would like to make a gift to *Rest Ministries* in the amount of _______ .
❑ I would like to partner with *Rest Ministries* & I pledge to give _______ . each month. * *Rest Ministries, Inc. is a 501(c)(3) nonprofit corporation. Your gift is tax-deductible.*
❑ I am interested in starting a HopeKeepers® Group for people who live with chronic illness or pain. ***You can find an information packet online.***

TOTAL Purchases/Gifts: .... $______________
FREE SHIPPING .... - 0 -
California residents add 7.75% to purchase (not donation).................. $_______
TOTAL: .... $_______

________ Check included made payable to Rest Ministries
________ Charge my: ❑ Visa ❑ Mastercard
Card # ____
Expiration date:______________
Cardholder's signature *(required)* ______________________________
Please print clearly.
Name: ____
Address: ____
City/State/Zip: _______________________________________
Phone number:_______________________________________
Email:____

❑ *Please sign me up for email updates from Rest Ministries.*